HANDBOOK ON CRITICAL SEXUAL ISSUES

Pope John Center
Task Force on Critical Sexual Issues

Carl A. Anderson, Esq.
Counsellor to the Under Secretary
U.S. Department of Health and
Human Services
Washington, D.C.

The Reverend Benedict M. Ashley,
O.P., Ph.D., S.T.M.
Professor of Moral Theology
Aquinas Institute of Theology
St. Louis, MO

Aphrodite Clamar, Ph.D.
Clinical Psychologist
New York, NY

The Reverend Francis X. Cleary, S.J.,
S.S.L., S.T.D.
Associate Professor,
Department of Theological Studies
St. Louis University, St. Louis, MO

†The Reverend John R. Connery,
S.J., S.T.D.
Cody Professor of Theology
Loyola University Chicago
Chicago, IL

K. Diane Daly, RN, NFPE
Co-Director, St. John's Mercy,
Natural Family Planning
Education and Research Center
St. Louis, MO

The Reverend Mark Dosh, S.T.M.,
Ph.D.
Pastor, St. Pius X Church
White Bear Lake
Ramsey County, MN

The Reverend Thomas P. Doyle, O.P.,
M.A., M.S., M.Ch.A., J.C.D.
Secretary
Apostolic Delegation
Washington, D.C.

The Reverend Joseph P. Gillespie,
O.P., D.Min.
Associate Professor of Pastoral
Theology
Aquinas Institute of Theology
St. Louis, MO

The Reverend John F. Harvey, OSFS,
M.A., S.T.D.
Professor of Moral Theology
Cluster of Independent Theological
Schools
Washington, D.C.

John F. Kippley, M.A.
Executive Director
Couple-to-Couple League
Cincinnati, OH

The Reverend Michael P.
McDonough, S.T.D.
Director of Social Ethics
Pope John Center
St. Louis, MO

James A. Monteleone, MD
Professor of Pediatrics
St. Louis University and Cardinal
Glennon Hospital
St. Louis, MO

Patricia L. Monteleone, MD
Professor of Pediatrics
St. Louis University School of
Medicine
St. Louis, MO

The Reverend Albert S.
Moraczewski, O.P., Ph.D.
Regional Director—Houston Office
Houston, TX

The.Reverend Thomas Morrow,
M.Div., Ed.D.
Psychologist/Psychotherapist
Catholic Charities of Diocese of
Brooklyn
Brooklyn, NY

Glenn W. Olsen, Ph.D.
Professor of History
University of Utah
Salt Lake City, UT

Pierre J. Payer, S.T.B., M.A., Ph.D.
Professor of Philosophy
Mount Saint Vincent University
Halifax, Nova Scotia

Konald A. Prem, MD
Chairman
Department of Obstetrics and
Gynecology
University of Minnesota School of
Medicine
Minneapolis, MN

Richard T.F. Schmidt, BS, MD
Director
Department of Obstetrics &
Gynecology
Good Samaritan Hospital, Cincinnati,
OH

Dermott Smith, MD
Professor of Psychiatry
St. Louis University School of
   Medicine
St. Louis, MO

HANDBOOK ON CRITICAL SEXUAL ISSUES

Revised Edition

Edited and revised by: Donald G. McCarthy, Ph.D.,
Edward J. Bayer, S.T.D,
John A. Leies, S.M., S.T.D.

The Pope John XXIII Center

Braintree, Massachusetts

Nihil Obstat:
Rev. James A. O'Donohoe, J.C.D.
Censor Deputatus

Imprimatur:
Bernard Cardinal Law
Archdiocese of Boston, June 14, 1989

Library of Congress Cataloging in Publication Data
Main entry under title:

Handbook on critical sexual issues / edited and revised by Donald G.
McCarthy, Edward J. Bayer, John A. Leies—Rev. ed.
p. cm.
Includes bibliographical references.
ISBN 0-935372-25-3
1. Sex—Religious aspects—Catholic Church. 2. Medical ethics.
3. Catholic church—Doctrines. I. McCarthy, Donald G. II. Bayer,
Edward J., 1930– . III. Leies, John A. IV. Pope John XXIII
Medical-Moral Research and Education Center.
HQ63.H36 1989
306.7—dc20   89-16252
                                                              CIP

Contents

Preface to the Second and Revised Edition

In the six years since the original edition was published in 1983, a number of developments in medical technology, as well as several official Church documents, have appeared and become subject of much public discussion. In addition, the editors have received a number of helpful comments, criticisms and suggestions based on the first edition, and wish to express here their gratitude to those who made them. In particular, they wish to thank the Reverend Francis Vollmecke, Ph.D., and the Reverend Leonard Glavin, O. F. M. Cap, Ph.D., professors of philosophy at the Pontifical College Josephinum for their assistance in rewriting the parts dealing with philosophical influences on contemporary American moral attitudes. The editors are also deeply grateful to Mrs. Jeanne L. Burke, who navigated this edition through months of preparation.

Finally, we wish to all the teachers, students, medical personnel, and others who will use this new revised edition an ever deepening share in the wisdom the Catholic community of faith can bring to the questions that face us in medical technology today, especially those arising from critical sexual issues.

Donald G. McCarthy, Ph.D.
Edward J. Bayer, S.T.D.
John A. Leies, S.M., S.T.D.

PART ONE

**Sexuality in Catholic Teaching:
Yesterday and Today**

Preview of
Chapter One

- The Bible proclaims the Christian vocation of love; Christianity teaches about sexual love because human sexuality is present in all human expressions of love.

- The Bible sees human creatures as ennobled by the sexual capacity God has given them for a conjugal relationship of loving intimacy and fruitfulness.

- The Old Testament portrays both the goodness of sexuality and marriage and the ways in which sin leads to selfish abuse of the gift of sexuality.

- The marriage covenant should reflect the love in God's covenant with His people; the two covenants mutually reveal each other.

- The interior gift of Christian holiness becomes the central concern in sexual morality throughout the New Testament.

- The New Testament teaches that marriage is not essential to a person's wholeness and happiness.

CHAPTER 1

Sexuality in the Bible

Love and Sexuality

"Beloved, if God has loved us so, we must have the same love for one another." (1 Jn. 4:11) Christianity proclaims for all people of all time a vocation of love.

Human persons do not love in a purely spiritual way as angels do. They love as bodily creatures who are physically present to one another. Furthermore, the human sexual identity as male or female provides the capacity for sexual intercourse as the supreme expression of bodily human love.

Christianity teaches about sexual love because human sexuality is present in all human expressions of love. Catholic Christianity recognizes one particular form of love, marriage, as a Sacrament, a sacred relationship in which the spouses are united in Christ when united in lasting mutual sexual love. *But both the Christian call to love and human sexuality itself embraces all persons, married or unmarried.*

In order to study critical sexual issues from the perspective of the Judeo-Christian tradition, this book considers human sexuality as it is understood and experienced in the Bible. Men and women of faith listen to the Word of God speaking about love and sexuality. The Bible is

3

called revelation because it reveals truth for God's people. Yet that truth can only be discovered through prayerful study and reflection. This chapter will initiate such an effort.

In the Beginning

The story of human sexual love begins in the Garden of Eden. Two accounts of human creation are found in the first two chapters of *Genesis*. The second account, which scholars consider the older one (Gn. 2:4–25), focuses on the relationship of *sexual intimacy* when "a man leaves his father and -mother and clings to his wife, and the two of them become one body." (v. 24)

The other account of human creation found in Gn. 1–2:4, focuses on human creation in the image of God with the divine blessing, "Be fruitful and multiply and fill the earth and subdue it." (v. 28) God not only created the first human persons, He also fashioned them into their complementary sexual identities as male and female and made possible the *relationship of sexual unity which can generate new human persons.*

The Bible thus sees human persons as only faith can see them—as creatures ennobled by the sexual capacity with which God has entrusted them. Yet the Biblical story of sin entering the world through God's first human creatures (Gn. Chap. 3) teaches that sin and selfishness will henceforth affect sexual behavior. The sexual relationship which offers promise of loving unity becomes, through sin, an occasion of exploitation, dominance, and manipulation.

Love and Sexuality in the Old Testament

Hence the Old Testament portrays both the goodness of sexuality and marriage and the ways in which sin leads to selfish abuse of the gift of sexuality. Throughout the books of the Old Testament, procreation, the fruitfulness of human sexual love, appears as a blessing while barrenness or sterility is a curse. The people of Israel rejoiced in parenthood. They gladly fulfilled God's promise: "God took Abram outside and said: 'Look up at the sky and count the stars, if you can. Just so', He added, ' shall your descendants be.'" (Gn. 15:5)

The Bible portrays instances of profoundly romantic love in the *Song of Songs* and in the story of Jacob who served his future father-in-law for seven years instead of paying a dowry for Rebecca, "yet they seemed to him but a few days because of his love for her." (Gn. 29:20) A newly married husband in Israel was exempt from military service and any public duty for one year, "to bring joy to the wife he has married." (Dt. 24:5)

Yet the Old Testament records the taking of multiple wives and concubines by some of the patriarchs. Evidently examples of misuse of sexuality among Israel's pagan neighbors affected the people of Israel. *The Law of Israel therefore explicitly forbade sexual misconduct including adultery, incest, homosexuality, rape, and bestiality.* (Lv. 20:10–21, Dt. 22:23–29, Gn. 18:20, and Ex. 22:18)

The marital roles and rights of women in Old Testament times were influenced by the prevailing cultural attitudes which did not admit full equality with men. The original *Genesis* creation account in chapters 2 and 3 had seemed to indicate equality of women and men in the "two in one flesh" image. Yet the Hebrew Law did not insist on full equality. For example, women were bound to unconditional fidelity to their husbands whereas Israelite men were apparently permitted multiple wives and concubines as long as they did not take another man's wife. In earlier Hebrew times, even fornication on the part of a man and adultery (at least if the woman involved were not married) were judged more leniently than these same sins on the part of a woman. The provisions made in Deuteronomy 21:10–14 for marriage with a captive woman, however, do recognize protection for such women unparalleled in the ancient world. Furthermore, the picture of the ideal wife in Proverbs 31:10–31 shows her with a great deal of authority and an extremely important economic role in the family structure.

The historical narratives of the Old Testament indicate a sense of responsibility before God for sexual behavior. For example, the story of Joseph and Potiphar's wife in Egypt presents Joseph's heroic resistance to adultery because this would be "great wickedness" and a "sin against God." (Gn. 39:9) Abraham misled Abimelech by describing his wife Sara as his sister because he suspected "there is no fear of God in this place." (Gn. 20:11) Abimelech, though, protested to God that he "did it in good faith and with clean hands." (Gn. 20:5)

Numerous Old Testament passages condemn prostitution, a widespread practice in the pagan religious rites and secular culture of the day. A legal text in Leviticus 19:29 tells fathers, "You shall not degrade your daughter by making a prostitute of her, else the land will become corrupt and full of lewdness." The Hebrew word translated by "degrade" regularly is used for the profane use of holy things or persons. This suggests a certain sacredness about the human sexual power and a moral responsibility of stewardship of it.

5

The prophets Amos and Jeremiah spoke out strongly against prostitution. (Am. 2:7, Jer. 5:7) The book of Sirach (written only 200 years before Jesus) reflects the firm sexual teaching of the final era of the Old Testament in a passage (9:3–9) which weaves together warnings against adultery, fornication, and prostitution in a way that indicates they are comparable kinds of sexual misbehavior. (Sirach 23:16–21 also condemns these sins and, many scholars think masturbation.[1]) In Sirach 42:10 a father's anxiety for his daughter includes a twofold concern: "While unmarried, lest she be seduced or, as a wife, lest she prove unfaithful."

Thus the Old Testament portrayal of human sexuality *begins in the innocence of the garden of Eden and then depicts a long history of sexual attitudes and behavior manifesting the tension and temptation arising from sin and selfishness.* The fact that marriage is intended by God to be a sacred relationship based on steadfast and undying love emerges gradually but dramatically from the Old Testament prophets, especially Hosea, Jeremiah, Isaiah, and Ezechiel. They used the image of human marriage as a sign or symbol of God's covenant of faithful love for His people. One theologian, Edward Schillebeeckx, speaks of a "reciprocal revelation" in which the prophets are "unveiling" both God's covenant and the marriage covenant.

The New Testament Law of Love

In the Old Testament period sexual attitudes and behavior were guided by the Law given to Moses. In the New Testament, however, Jesus Christ becomes the supreme teacher of morality and the source of salvation. St. Peter referred to both Jews and Gentiles at the Council of Jerusalem when he said, "Our belief is rather that we are saved by the favor of the Lord Jesus and so are they." (Acts 15:11) *Hence the New Testament emphasizes the interior holiness proclaimed and provided by Jesus.*

In dialogue with the scribe in chapter 12 of Mark, Jesus taught this interior holiness which can be called the "law of love" and presented it as the love of God and neighbor. This love led the penitent woman to forgiveness when Jesus said of her in Luke's gospel, "I tell you, that is why her many sins are forgiven—because of her great love." (Lk. 7:47) Jesus proposed His doctrine of love in John: "Such as my love has been for you, so must your love be for each other. This is how all will know you for my disciples: your love for one another." (Jn. 13:34–35)

St. Paul taught the Christian doctrine of love as Christ's gift of interior holiness. He wrote to the Romans that "The love of God has been poured out in our hearts through the Holy Spirit who has been given to us." (Rom. 5:5) To the Galatians he wrote, "It is in the spirit that we eagerly await the justification we hope for, and only faith can yield it." (Gal. 5:5)

St. Paul insisted on the interior presence of the Spirit as essential to holiness: "If anyone does not have the Spirit of Christ, he does not belong to Christ." (Rom. 8:9). The Spirit's presence brings the Christian new life and a new relationship to God: "All who are led by the Spirit of God are sons of God. You did not receive a spirit of slavery leading you back into fear, but a spirit of adoption through which we cry out, 'Abba,' that is, 'Father.'" (Rom. 8:14–15).

This vision of Christian holiness becomes the central concern in sexual morality throughout the New Testament. St. Paul summarized it after vigorously opposing prostitution in the First Epistle to the Corinthians.

> Shun lewd conduct. Every other sin a man commits is outside his body, but the fornicator sins against his own body. You must know that your body is a temple of the Holy Spirit, who is within—the Spirit you have received from God. (1 Cor. 6:18–19)

Hence, in summary, the Old Testament covenant of salvation was replaced in the New Testament by the new covenant of Jesus Christ. Jesus proclaimed unselfish love as the centerpiece of human life. This kind of love comes from the abiding interior presence of the Spirit. *Those who accept this gift are called to manifest it by sexual behavior which respects the authentic role of sexuality in human relationships.*

The Continuity of Moral Teaching

The New Testament emphasis on holiness and authentic love is applicable to the basic framework of sexual morality already taught in the Old Testament. Marriage becomes a relationship modeled on Christ's love for the Church. (Eph. 5:25–31) Adultery is rejected (Mk. 7:22, Mt. 15:19, 1 Cor. 6:9), as are adulterous desires and intentions. (Mt. 5:28) It is quite possible also that Jesus warns specifically against masturbation.[2]

The internal holiness which accords with the presence of the Spirit leads St. Paul to oppose even conversation which suggests sexual immorality: "As for lewd conduct or promiscuousness or lust of any sort, let them not even be mentioned among you; your holiness forbids this. Nor

7

should there be any obscene, silly, or suggestive talk; all that is out of place." (Eph. 5:3–4)

Jesus Himself described sin as internal corruption or "wicked designs" which lead to a whole series of evil actions including fornication and adultery: "Wicked designs come from the deep recesses of the heart: acts of fornication, theft, murder, adulterous conduct, greed, maliciousness, deceit, sensuality, envy, blasphemy, arrogance, an obtuse spirit. All these evils come from within and render a man impure." (Mk. 7:21–23)

This "list of vices" from Mark's gospel corresponds with St. Paul's listing of the works of the "flesh" in the epistle to the Galatians. (5:16–21) Some of these actions, like deceit, envy, and arrogance, are not primarily bodily actions. Hence, the "flesh" does not necessarily mean bodily activity, and St. Paul is not specifically condemning sexual activity when he condemns actions "of the flesh." What are condemned are selfish manifestations of sexuality, such as adultery and fornication.

Modern Biblical scholars have discussed the exact meaning of the Greek word *porneia* which is sometimes translated "immorality" and sometimes "fornication." It surely includes sexual intercourse with prostitutes, whether in pagan religious rituals or in the traditional commercial bargain. Does it also include sexual intercourse between unmarried persons who are in love and perhaps even engaged? Catholic teaching includes these sexual relations as fornication, although the situation may not have presented itself very frequently in New Testament times. *St. Paul would seem to have rejected such premarital activity as immoral, especially in 1 Cor. 7:2 where he writes, "To avoid immorality (porneia), every man should have his own wife and every woman her own husband."*

The New Testament opposition to selfish sexual behavior and to sexual relations outside the marital relationship leads implicitly to a fuller recognition of women's dignity, despite the influence of cultural discrimination. In fact, Jesus was protecting women from exploitation when He took a stronger stand against divorce than Moses. The doctrine in which Jesus proclaimed that a man committed adultery when he divorced his wife in favor of another woman obviously presumed a lifelong fidelity of the husband to one wife in contrast to the practices of some Old Testament figures. (Mt. 19:3–12)

St. Paul, while teaching wives to be submissive to their husbands, does proclaim a mutuality and equality in marital love. "Husbands should love their wives as they do their own bodies," he writes. "He who loves his wife loves himself." (Eph. 5:28) Wives are equal to their husbands in having a right to the sexual expression of married love. (1 Cor. 7:4) Paul also provided the clearest statement in the New Testa-

8

ment of the equal dignity of women with men when he wrote to the Galatians: "There does not exist among you Jew or Greek, slave or freeman, male or female. All are one in Christ Jesus." (Gal. 3:28)

The concern for the equal dignity of men and women highlighted here leads to a concluding theme on this subject of sexuality in the Bible, the personalism of New Testament teaching.

Personalism in the New Testament

In contrast to the Old Testament, the New Testament makes clear provision for a personal and fully acceptable decision to remain unmarried. Jesus told His disciples in chapter 19 of Matthew, "Some there are who have freely renounced sex for the sake of God's reign. Let him accept this teaching who can." Some few scholars think Jesus was not referring here to celibacy, as most interpreters believe, but rather to the obligation of a person who is married but separated from his or her spouse.

In either case Jesus, and St. Paul after Him, clearly recognize that marriage is not essential to a person's wholeness and happiness. In Mark 12:25 Jesus explains to the Sadducees that marriage is only a temporary condition of a world which is passing away.

This doctrine need not imply a downgrading of marriage or a suggestion that human sexual activity is inherently corrupt or degrading. St. Paul recognizes the call to marriage or to celibacy as a gift accorded to individuals. "Given my preference, I should like you to be as I am," he wrote to the Corinthians. "Still, each one has his gift from God, one this and another that." (1 Cor. 7:7)

St. Paul also recognized that married persons should not deprive one another of conjugal activity "unless perhaps by mutual consent for a time." (1 Cor. 7:1–7) In the first letter to Timothy the goodness of marriage is affirmed, perhaps in opposition to exaggerated views of the merits of celibacy (1 Tim. 4:3–4). The letter to the Hebrews exhorts that marriage be "honored in every way" (Heb. 13:4). The first epistle to Timothy assumes that in those first days of the Church bishops and deacons will be married. (1 Tim. 3:2 & 12)

A clarification of the role of sexuality in human life can, however, be found underlying the New Testament option to remain unmarried. As noted in the introduction to this chapter, human sexuality is present in *all* human expressions of love. New Testament personalism emphasizes that each human person must make a personal choice between the unique vocation of marital love and alternate vocations which manifest human love in a non-genital way.

9

This suggests that the traditional virtue of chastity should be seen as a quality to be cultivated by both married and unmarried persons. For married persons chastity will offer strength and guidance in their authentic and unselfish expressions of sexual love, including the unique and supreme expression which is marital intercourse.

Unmarried persons are still sexual persons by nature and still called by Christ to the holiness of unselfish love of God and neighbor. *For them chastity will offer strength and guidance in the proper expressions of love for persons of the same and the opposite sex, while foregoing marital intercourse which presumes a marital covenant.*

Thus chastity becomes the practical guiding virtue for Christians seeking to express love for one another in accord with the New Testament law of love. As a virtue it is cultivated within the heart of each person, an interior disposition which becomes one of the "fruits" of the Spirit, along with love, joy, and peace. (Gal. 5:22)

Discussion Questions

1. Why is Christianity concerned with human sexuality?
2. How did Old Testament attitudes toward human sexual behavior differ from modern attitudes?
3. Does the New Testament change the basic Old Testament framework of sexual morality?
4. How does the New Testament relate sex and love?
5. Does St. Paul condemn sexual activity when he condemns actions "of the flesh?"
6. How does the free decision to marry or remain single reflect personalism in the New Testament?

Notes

1. This passage mentions "three kinds of sins of impurity, with increasing degrees of gravity: solitary sins (16), fornication (17), and adultery (18–21)". The *New American Bible* (New York, 1970: Catholic Book Co.), p. 792 (Old Testament section), at bottom of the page for Sirach 23:16.

2. John P. Meier, *The Vision of Matthew* (New York, 1979: Paulist), p. 246, note 21, commenting on Jesus' remark about "if your right hand is a scandal to you," (Mt. 5:27–30): "Rabbinic texts also speak of adultery of the heart, hand, and eye; adultery of the hand may refer to masturbation, and this may be the meaning in the Matthean context."

Preview of Chapter Two

● Early Church teaching about sexuality was not proclaimed in a unified way by Pope and Bishops in Councils, but by individual bishops acting locally largely on their own initiative. This teaching sometimes lacked depth and balance which latter development would correct.

● At least seven different factors can be cited for the incompleteness and, at times deficiency of much early Christian thought about sexuality.

● A tension existed in the first centuries of the Church between an involvement view and an abandonment view of the world. There was a consequent tendency to emphasize the dangers and liabilities of marriage.

● Augustine defended marriage even though he saw it partially as a restraint for harnessing sexual desire toward its only worthy purpose: the procreation of children.

● Medieval theologians began taking a more positive view of marriage and the use of marital intercourse, although the handbooks for confessors still reflected somewhat the negative bias apparent in writings of previous centuries.

CHAPTER 2

Early and Medieval Catholic Teaching on Sexuality

The Church in our own 20th century speaks clearly in her official teaching regarding human sexuality. She clearly insists, for instance, on the goodness of genital actions which express a married couple's acceptance of their belonging uniquely and exclusively to each other, and of their vocation to give life to children.

Consistent with this position and with equal clarity, the Church repudiates as beneath human dignity all genital actions which are premarital, extra-marital, masturbatory, homosexual, or contraceptive. Even those who differ with her official teaching on these issues recognize, often with irritation, that the position is clear.

Balance and Depth Come Slowly

The Church's position regarding these issues has been clear from her beginnings. Throughout her first 1200 years, however, her teaching about sexual activity was different from her teaching today in two important ways. First, *it was not disseminated with one voice* by councils of bishops such as we have today or by a statement of the Pope to the world-wide Church; instead, this and all other moral teaching had to be garnered from writings of many scattered individual bishops and other Christian leaders and from the way lay people tried to live. Second, *teaching on sexuality lacked depth and balance.* Let us examine each difference in turn.

One of the most important sources of information from which we can garner information about the early Church's teachings on sexuality is a group of books called the *Penitentials.*[1] Written by Irish monks as early as the 6th century, these small booklets basically did nothing but list standard penances for various kinds of sins, including sexual ones. They did not, for instance, explain in detail *why* certain actions were evil. These booklets were widely used and quite rapidly found their way to England and the continent. *All this happened without any corporate action by the bishops and without the initiative of the Pope.*

The second difference, a lack of depth and balance, was unavoidable: *It was going to take centuries to understand fully and deeply the many complex aspects of sexual life within marriage,* and many generations of prayer, experience and contemplation to fit them all together in a balanced way.[2]

It was obvious to the early Christians, for example, that sexual intercourse is in some way inextricably tied to having children. Did that mean, then, that a man had a right to have children by his wife, even though he had fallen into a sinful attitude of cruelty and hatred towards her?

It was obvious also that a man and wife are called to love one another. Did that mean that the physical conjugal act, therefore, was planned by God to be an *expression* of this love? Or was that act *only* a bodily mechanism for producing a pregnancy?

These and similar questions seem not to have entered the minds of many early bishops and Christian writers. Or, if these questions did enter their minds, many religious teachers—and sometimes several generations of them—came up with incomplete and unbalanced answers. On certain points a few writers even went clearly into error by actually contradicting the universal teaching of the Church on some points.

The Root of Inadequate Answers

The incompleteness and even deficiency of much early Christian thought about sexuality was due to a number of factors.[3]

1) A PRESUMPTION OF SOME CHRISTIANS THAT JESUS IN-

TENDED TOTAL SEXUAL ABSTENTION TO BE A GOAL FOR ALL HIS FOLLOWERS. A misguided reverence for Christ and his personal life of celibacy led many Christians to conclude that only "weak Christians" were exempt from a celibate life; to encourage total abstention from sexual relations even within marriage itself; and to discourage the widowed from marrying again.

2) A PRESUMPTION THAT THE END OF THE WORLD WAS SOON TO COME. Early Christians were conscious that, in this matter, "no one knows the day or the hour." (Mark 13:32) Many presumed, however, that the end would be not long in coming. They wondered, therefore, about the wisdom of marrying and having a family if the Second Coming of Christ were a matter of perhaps only a few years or even a few months.

3) A SINCERE BUT OVERSIMPLIFIED REVERENCE FOR THE JEWISH SCRIPTURES. This reverence often led early Christians to govern their lives by certain Old Testament laws regarding sexual matters. They did not stop to think that many of these laws were merely God's teaching devices to impress on the Jewish people the special holiness of life and of the sexual sources of life. Thus, for example, men experiencing an accidental loss of semen in their sleep, or women experiencing the normal flow of menstrual blood could not join in the worship in the Temple until they had fulfilled certain prescribed rituals, such as ablutions, sacrifices, or the like. Intercourse during menstruation was forbidden. Many early Christians presumed that such norms applied to themselves.

4) A REVULSION AT PAGAN IMMORALITY. The pain, chaos, and ugliness of pagan sexual excesses in the Roman world were obvious, as were their effects on the crumbling societal life within the Empire. Moreover, many Christians reacted against this decadence with special fervor because they themselves had lived degrading lives before their conversion to Christ in Baptism.

5) THE PREDOMINANCE OF PLATO'S IDEAS ABOUT THE BODY. The Greek philosopher Plato, who wrote around 350 B.C., had taught that only the soul was the human person, and that the way to become more human was to escape the influences of one's body. By the year 100 A.D., people everywhere in the Roman world were taking Plato's views for granted as valid and true. Christians too were influenced by Plato, and for many centuries did not call his ideas into question. These views inevitably led to a less than enthusiastic evaluation of sexual desire and sexual union, even within marriage.

6) THE THOUGHT OF THE STOICS. Philosophers known in history as "The Stoics" greatly prized the laws of nature for the physi-

cal beauty and order they produce. This made their ideas attractive, not only to pagans who saw moral chaos swamping the Roman Empire in the first century, but also to Christians who believed that God is the Creator of nature's order. Unfortunately, the Stoics also despised affection, emotion, physical pleasure, and dependence on other persons. As a result, they could not see that sexual intercourse was designed to express marital love. They saw only that intercourse could produce a beautiful physical effect, namely, the conception of a child. Many Christians presumed that on this point the Stoics were correct.

7) THE LIMITATIONS OF EARLY BIOLOGICAL SCIENCE. Although some good beginnings in science had been made by men like Aristotle, little had been achieved by way of scientific understanding of our human reproductive processes. Strange theories abounded; for example, some people believed that intercourse during menstruation would produce deformed or leprous children. Such misunderstandings sometimes entered into Christians' considerations of sexual morality.

A Double Mind About Life In The World

Many of the above-mentioned factors converged in the minds of Christians of the first century and long afterwards to create what one might call a "double-mind," that is, a push and pull of two seemingly contradictory attitudes towards anything about life in this world, including sexuality.

The first of these seemingly contradictory attitudes was, *"Be involved in this present world in order to make it more a reflection of God's goodness."* It was evident to Christians that a great deal of good came from this present world. The Roman Empire, for all its failings, did establish much order and maintained an important kind of peace. There was, moreover, an obvious natural fulfillment in marriage and children. More important for Christians, their Jewish heritage proclaimed the world a blessing from God, and that blessing included marriage. Finally, Jesus himself had seemed to take delight in many things of this world; witness His actions at the wedding feast of Cana.

The second attitude was, *"Have as little as possible to do with this world, for it only keeps you from union with Christ."* This view, too, had a certain validity. Several devout groups of Jews before and during the time of Jesus had abandoned the life of Jerusalem and its Temple to establish austere communities out in the desert near the Dead Sea. Jesus himself

15

had refused to accept any earthly power. He also had lived a celibate life, and commended it to others.

There was, then, something true to Jesus in both of these attitudes. It must be admitted, however, that in many ways the second one largely dominated Christian minds for many centuries.

Some Christians even theorized that human sexuality might indeed be a kind of deformity of the body resulting from Original Sin. If the first human beings had not sinned, they reasoned, this unfortunate arrangement called sexual intercourse would not be part of human life.

Such an extremist theory was typical of what one might call "the abandonment view" among many Christian writers. They believed we must abandon worldly pursuits, including sexual activity within marriage. This mentality survived in various ways through the centuries, and even exists in some degree today.

Doubts Raised About "The Abandonment View"

As early as the year 200 A.D., however, several prominent Christian thinkers began to question the widespread "abandonment view" and its discouragement of an active sexual life within marriage. One Bishop, Clement of Alexandria in Egypt, pointed out what many Christians had forgotten: that *marriage, like earthly possessions, is not just allowed, but is to be enjoyed as God's good gift.* The Christian is not to flee the world, but to use it according to reason. *Marriage and celibacy are not two grades of perfection,* but two parallel states of life freely willed by God for different persons, and freely chosen by them in obedience to His call.

Tertullian, also writing in the second century, described the beauty of marriage between Christians in his inspiring *Letter to My Wife.*

" . . . two who are one in hope, one in religion. They are brother and sister, both servants of the same Master. Nothing divides them, either in flesh or in spirit."

At about the same time, Origen taught that God intended the physical conjugal act to be an image of the spiritual love between Christ and the Church.

Eusebius of Caesarea, who died in 340 A.D., saw the celibate life, for all its privileged calling, as an exception to God's plan that most people marry and be active in restoring a damaged world to God's image.

Most of these same writers, however, did at least occasionally show traces of the more pessimistic "abandonment view." Especially persistent was the idea that sexual activity within marriage was a "concession to

16

weakness" (Clement of Alexandria) or a "protection against fornication."
(John Chrysostom) And always lurking in the background was the basic
position of Plato: the living human body is not really part of the true
human being.

Erroneous Starting Points[4]

Several mistaken attitudes led to many early Christians' hesitation
about accepting an active sexual life as a valuable service to God.

It is clear now, for instance, that *one of their mistakes was to concentrate
on the dangers and liabilities that come with marriage.* Concentration on problems, real enough as these were, kept many Christian thinkers from
fully appreciating the good things which God originally created in marriage, and which have never been lost.

*Another mistake was to treat marriage as an option only for "the weak"
Christian,* while assuming that total sexual abstinence was meant for "the
strong" Christian.

It is true that, from the words and example of Jesus, one can say
that *in some sense* celibacy is superior to marriage. But this does not
mean that celibacy is *in every sense* superior to marriage. For only in marriage can two human beings celebrate the way God has made them as
male and female by using their genital powers to express both their true
love and their call to give life to children.

It is true also that *in some sense* marriage does shield some persons
from falling into sexual sins. But it is true also that many married persons would be capable of living chastely outside of marriage. Nonetheless, God does, for reasons of his own, call them to marriage. Moreover,
marriage can itself be an occasion of sins, such as an economic, psychological, physical or even sexual "using" of one's partner as if he or she
were not a person, but a thing.

Augustine's Praise of Marriage[5]

The most influential writer of the first 1200 years of the Church's
life was St. Augustine, who died in 430 A.D. Though burdened by many
of the biases already mentioned, *Augustine made a highly intelligent effort to
see and defend the goods which God has created in marriage.*

He was careful to defend a kind of superiority for celibacy, while
insisting that celibacy or any other external way of life did not make a
person a better Christian. Only charity, he insisted,—love of God and of
one's neighbor in God—could do that. And charity, he points out, is not

17

only present, but also sometimes more outstanding in the lives of the married than of celibates. Augustine also denounced the theory that human sexual differentiation, desires, and activities were a kind of deformity resulting from Original Sin. Beginning to break with extremist versions of Plato's thought, Augustine recognized that bodily life is a part of the human person. He recognized also that lifelong faithfulness in marriage was the highest form of human friendship. On occasion (but *only* on occasion) he even mentioned that sexual intercourse may very well be intended by God to be itself an expression of the love between husband and wife. Finally, Augustine pointed out how the procreating of children and the love through which this happens is an image in human flesh of the fruitful and eternal love between Christ and the Church.

Augustine's Ethical Positions

Despite his magnificent defense of marriage, however, Augustine preached a severely demanding ethic for the married. Unlike certain non-Christian writers, he saw sexuality not as a *bad* animal, but as a *wild* one needing to be restrained within marriage. Marriage alone offered this restraint by harnessing sexual desire towards achieving its only worthy purpose: the procreation of children. As a matter of fact, he taught that *only a conscious desire to have a child could justify a couple's act of intercourse.*

It is a commonplace observation that Augustine's rigorist attitudes can undoubtedly be traced to his experience of the breakdown of Roman society. Widespread sexual depravity was playing its part in this breakdown, and Augustine knew that depravity only too well: he himself had lived in it for 33 years before his conversion to Christ.

Gnostics and Christian Groups

Christian thinkers such as Augustine were struggling to spell out the good things in marriage. At the same time one very influential non-Christian religious group, the gnostics, was holding that the material world, including the human body, could only be the work of a god who is evil. Only purely spiritual beings, such as our souls, are the work of a god who is good. For the gnostics and other similar groups, sexual intercourse was the worst of all sins, for it simply fashioned one more evil "prison," that is, a body in which some unfortunate soul would be entrapped for years. Some gnostics tried to re-interpret the new Christian

18

religion in order to promote their ideas. Influenced by such reinterpretation, a few Christian groups came to despise the human body and its sexuality as evil. No longer truly Christian, these groups nonetheless often attempted to retain some Christian elements. Various strains of gnosticism continued to appear in sects separate from the Catholic Church as late as the 7th century and resurfaced even as late as the 12th century in a group called the Albigensians.

Other groups which were not gnostic nonetheless broke off from the Catholic Church because they insisted on a rigorist view of sexuality which the Church would not accept. The great Tertullian wound up outside the Church partly because of his insistence that a second marriage for a widow was adultery.

The Middle Ages: Christians Begin to Think More Deeply About Marriage

For the first thousand years of the Church's life, as noted above, the teachings on marriage and sexuality were scattered throughout thousands of homilies, theological treatises on other subjects, and guidelines for imposing penances. In the 12th century, however, for the first time whole books began to appear treating marriage extensively.

The first people to produce in-depth treatises on marriage were the canonists, that is, clergymen who served as lawyers on Church courts. The canonists were primarily concerned with settling cases where someone claimed that a marriage had never been valid or that it had never been consummated. As a result, their treatises had a tendency to rely almost entirely on the legal precedents of the previous centuries of the Church's life. *The canonists made little effort to go to the Scriptures to understand more deeply what marriage is.*

Theologians such as Peter Lombard, Albert the Great, Bonaventure, and Scotus, working precisely from the Scriptures and using the methods of logical thought developed by philosophers such as Aristotle, also produced whole treatises on marriage and sexual activity. Unfortunately, they tended to accept without question most of the theories which the canonists had developed to explain the decisions of Church courts. Thus, instead of Church law following a deeper understanding of Christian doctrine, *the understanding of doctrine tended to depend upon accepted practice in Church law.* Although this situation sometimes produced a rather shallow theology, both theology and canon law benefited from the new studies.

The great collection of thousands of Church laws and judicial decisions by Gratian around the year 1100 A.D. shows some attempt to critique the legal opinions of the past in light of a deeper understanding of the teachings of Christ, while theology itself was stimulated to further its own work by the new and intense work of the canonists. Peter Lombard, in his treatise *The Sentences,* laid the basis for the magnificent work of Thomas Aquinas (1225–1274) who explored in depth the variety of opinions expressed on marriage from the beginning of the Church.

Aquinas often rejected venerable opinions even of sainted early writers. Citing the theory that our sexual desires and actions are a kind of deformity resulting from Original Sin, Aquinas says bluntly of certain Church Fathers, "In saying this they spoke unreasonably."

Aquinas accepts the common teaching that in *justice,* that is by a kind of *contract* between them, a man and wife owe it to each other to remain together for life. He notes, however, that *they must remain together even more so because of the love* into which they have freely entered. This love, he then remarks, is expressed both *by living as a family unit* and *by the conjugal embrace of intercourse.*[6]

Other theologians, such as the Franciscan school represented by Nicholas Oresme in the 14th century and Martin Le Maistre in the 15th, were beginning to see that the desire for sexual pleasure, and not only the desire to conceive a child, could be enough reason to make sexual intercourse licit. With Thomas, they also recognized that the Old Testament rules about menstruation, the inadvertent loss of semen, and the conjugal act itself were not binding on Christians. For instance, while the new theologians continued to regard conjugal relations during menstruation as illicit they explicitly based this point of teaching not on the Old Testament, but on the opinion commonly held in their day that deformed or leprous offspring could result from such relations.

The lessons taught the people as they received the sacraments were perhaps as important on the practical pastoral level as were the scholarly discussions of the theologians. On the one hand, a new type of handbook for priest-confessors, the *Summa Confessorum,* was a distinct improvement over the old *Penitentials* of the 6th century. Unfortunately, however, these handbooks still reflected much of the negative bias of previous ages against marriage and sexuality. On the other hand, *the wedding liturgy presented the goodness of marriage and its physical union* so clearly as to enable an honest Christian couple to make love without scrupulous concern over the details of their motivation and the pleasure they would experience.

Conclusion

The work of demolishing exaggerated hesitations about marriage and of deepening the Church's appreciation of God's gift of sexuality had begun, but much more remained to be done. While events of later centuries threw more obstacles into the path of understanding, the same events also raised new questions which have enabled the Church to see more clearly than ever just how wise the Lord is to have made us in His image by making us male and female.

Discussion Questions

1. Does the Catholic Church claim to have understood clearly all the implications of the teaching of Christ regarding sexuality? Or does she claim to have progressed through the centuries in understanding this teaching?
2. What are five ideas which early Christians presumed to be true regarding sexuality, without actually seeing whether they were necessarily connected with the teaching of Christ?
3. What two contradictory attitudes towards the world did early Christians have to wrestle with? Was either of these attitudes totally erroneous?
4. Give six points in which St. Augustine defended marriage.
5. A Polish theologian, Karol Wojtyla, later Pope John Paul II, wrote in 1960, "There is no reason to hold that sexual intercourse must necessarily have conception as its end. . . . We cannot therefore demand of spouses that they positively desire to procreate on every occasion when they have intercourse." How does this compare with Augustine's teachings?
6. Which theologians began to explore the conjugal act as an expression of love between spouses?

Notes

1. Bieler, L. (ed.) *The Irish Penitentials*. Scriptores Latini Hiberniae, Dublin, 1963.

2. Schillebeeckx, E., *Marriage: Human Reality and Saving Mystery*. New York, 1965. See especially Volume I, part 2.

3. Noonan, John, *Contraception: A History of Its Treatment by Catholic Theologians and Canonists*. Cambridge, Mass., 1965. For a critique of some of Noonan's points see Parmisano, footnote 6 below.

It should be noted that Noonan, at least until very recently and perhaps even now, advocates revising the traditional Church condemnation of artificial contraception. Some judge his work biased on this issue. Be that as it may, the present editors believe that he offers a wealth of useful information and documentation which can scarcely can be found elsewhere in English on Christian attitudes towards contraception. Near the end of his book, Noonan even notes particularly that one key element is present consistently throughout 1700 years of Catholic belief and teaching:

The act of coitus is sacred, is invested with a nonhuman immunity. It is *sacramental* for Christians and non-Christians alike. Why is it thus? Because by

21

means of it God permits two human beings to join in the creative task of producing human life. The unique power of this act is such that every instance of its exercise must be treated reverently, as one would a sacrament. The criticisms [against contraception] based on the function of the biological system, the analogies drawn from animal behavior, even the arguments [favoring contraception] showing that to absolutize this value [of procreation] destroys other marital values—all these miss the point. *The act is absolute, interference with its natural function is immoral, because it is the act from which life begins.*

It would be possible to read the teaching of theologians and canonists, popes and bishops, for over seventeen hundred years, as embodying this position. To do so would require isolating a single strand of the teaching from other reasons and treating it, abstracted from all contexts, as dispositive of the morality of any act which, in the exercise of coitus, "intentionally deprives it of its natural power and strength". *(ibid., pp. 530–31, emphasis added)*

Curiously, Noonan then drops the point. As it turned out, this "single strand of the teaching" is precisely what Pope Paul VI in the encyclical *Humanae Vitae,* three years after Noonan's book, and Pope John Paul II in his 1981 *Familiaris Consortio* and other teachings, take up and develop in a highly personalist way. (See chapter 5 of this book.) They point to this *sacred, quasi-sacramental* aspect of the conjugal act as, in itself, decisive for rejecting contraception as an immoral assault against that act. Thus they develop the very point which, for some reason, Noonan's book leaves undeveloped: that the conjugal act must be a *sign* or *expression* of the couple's dedication to one another in a love which is precisely *sexual.* In other words, their *conjugal act* must be *authentically* a human sexual act—open to whatever new life God might want to create out of it. Any "sexual" act which, in its very physical structure, can express only a defiant NO to any new life God might want to create is simply no longer authentically a human sexual act. It is, these popes teach, simply beneath our human dignity.

Equally curiously, Noonan draws from this "single strand" of the traditional teaching one conclusion which, it seems to the present editors, is obviously false: that "the use of the pill" would be legitimate because [unlike condoms, diaphragms, mutual masturbation, etc.] it leaves the "sacred" and "sacramental" physical structure of the conjugal act intact! Such a conclusion, of course, ignores the obvious fact that a sacrament is made *false* even if the *physical, visible* elements are used, but the *internal intention* of those using them is against the very meaning of the sacrament. At any rate, whatever its deficiencies, we believe that readers will find his book highly instructive.

4. Daniélou, Jean *The Origins of Latin Christianity.* especially pp. 356–357.

5. Brown, Peter, *Augustine of Hippo: A biography.* Berkley, 1969.

6. Parmisano, F. "Love and Marriage in the Middle Ages, I and II," *New Blackfriars.* 50 (1968–69) pp. 599–608 and 649–660.

Preview of Chapter Three

• After nominalism undermined the medieval system of thought named Thomism after St. Thomas Aquinas, the Reformation led to a renewal of Catholic theology.

• But in moral theology, or Christian ethics, more attention was paid to solving individual cases than to a systematic study of human nature and moral activity.

• Popes like Alexander VII and Innocent XI began speaking out on sexual issues in the 17th century. In the 18th, St. Alphonsus Liguori became the most prominent moral theologian of that period.

• In the 20th century, new emphasis was placed on the marital act as intended to express conjugal love in its totality, including its openness both to one's spouse and to whatever new life God might want to give from it. In 1930 Pope Pius XI wrote the first encyclical addressed to the whole Church on sexuality.

• Pope Pius XII addressed offical teaching on contraception and related issues in response to questions raised after World War II. He explicitly approved the use of natural family planning when avoiding a pregnancy for serious reasons.

CHAPTER 3

Catholic Sexual Teaching Before Vatican II

How does God expect us to lead our sexual lives? Why has he made us as male and female? Are there some sexual actions truly beneath us? And if so, why?

The Catholic Church has believed from her beginning that she has an obligation to answer such questions out of her deep knowledge of Jesus Christ. She is not always ready, however, to answer them at the highest levels of her teaching authority, namely that of the Pope or the bishops united in a Plenary Council. For sometimes long periods, she remains confident that her people are getting a truly Christian view of sexuality and marriage from the Bible, the words of the wedding rite, and the example and instruction of their families and pastors. The Church also depends upon the work of experts whom we call theologians, as they try to explain accurately and deeply the meaning, the reasons, and the implications of the teaching which the Church upholds in the name of Christ.

With very few exceptions, the Church saw no need for teaching on sexuality from her highest levels of authority prior to the sixteenth century. Around 1049, Pope Leo IX commended St. Peter Damian for his writings against permissive attitudes towards masturbation, homosexuality, and bestiality. At the same time, the Pope cautioned against cruelty and needlessly harsh judgement towards sinners. The Fourth Lateran Council (1215) defended sexual life in marriage as good, against the heresy of the Albigensians who taught that all sexual activity was evil. The Council of Florence (1439) echoed previous Councils' teaching that the marriage bond, once consummated sexually, was as unbreakable as the love of Christ and the Church. These few examples, however, are all one finds of teaching at the highest level touching on sexual matters.[1]

Theologians also sought to present not only what the Church teaches, but why as noted previously, prior to 1500, St. Thomas Aquinas, Nicholas Oresme, and Martin Le Maistre had begun exploring how the conjugal act is not only a bodily mechanism for conceiving a child, but at the same time an expression of dedicated love.[2] *St. Thomas' approach, called Thomism, was to seek out what is most fundamental about being a Christian, being a human, or being at all.* To achieve this, he used a *careful analysis* of what is found in the *Bible. Church teaching,* and our *experience of the human person.* St. Thomas believed that careful analysis could successfully bring out truths which might otherwise escape our attention. *Only a grasp of these fundamental truths would enable us to make decisions worthy of human beings and Christians.*

Unfortunately, by 1500 most theologians had entirely abandoned Thomas' approach in every area of theology, including ethical teaching, and embraced a philosophy called Nominalism. Nominalists taught that anything we say about the most basic questions of life or about the teachings of Christ are mere words (in Latin, *nomina*) which can never begin to reflect the truth.[3]

Catholic versus Protestant

By the year 1500, then, many theologians had lost confidence in their being able to say anything of real service to the Church. With the collapse of serious theological work came also a widespread confusion about doctrine, a weakening in morality even among the clergy, and superstition. Moreover, kings and nobility were making new and often successful attempts to get the Church under their control.

25

As a result of all this, a religious rebellion broke out in Germany under Martin Luther. Within 20 years, Christians in many countries were no longer Catholic. Luther and other Protestant leaders rejected the authority structure of the Church, some of the sacraments, and some basic points of Catholic belief.

In reaction, Catholic theologians woke up to what a mistake it had been for previous generations to have abandoned the profound approach of St. Thomas Aquinas. They returned to his method in order to clarify and defend the doctrines attacked by the Protestants.

The one thing the Catholic theologians did not have to defend, however, was the moral teaching of the Church, for Protestants generally retained this entirely. *Thus Catholic theologians did not turn their talents and their renewed Thomistic approach to a clarification of the foundations of sexual morality.*

Courses for Priest-Confessors

After the Council of Trent (1545–1563), however, a number of brilliant theologians did turn their talents to *re-establishing a disciplined moral life* in the Catholic Church.[4] Their strategy was to provide courses to train priests especially well for the hearing of confessions. In 1600, John Azor published the first *Institutiones* or instructions for confessors, and other writers quickly followed suit. On some points, however, authors could not agree among themselves, and the next 150 years saw a number of heated controversies.

Unfortunately, the authors of the various *Institutiones* did *not* apply the methods of St. Thomas thoroughly to the most important *sources* of moral teaching, namely the Bible and the constant doctrine of the Church. *Instead* they concentrated on individual moral *problems*, that is, the cases a confessor might come up against. This method was called *casuistry* or the *study of cases*. Casuistry would try to see how one moral case differed from another and required a different response.

Thus, for instance, confessors came up against cases of women who had been raped and immediately afterwards sought to get rid of the semen in order to escape impregnation. Some authors saw this as morally equivalent to a husband's interrupting the conjugal act by ejaculating outside the vagina in order to avoid pregnancy. Other authors said it was an entirely different "case," and that the rape victims were correct in what they did. Neither side, however, went into the true nature of the conjugal act as presented in the Bible or in the common teaching of the Church. Instead, both sides based their argument on primitive erroneous biological theories of the time. They also concentrated on the interplay of various "laws" or "commandments" of God which in a given "case" seemed to clash with one another. They tried to decide which "law" or "commandment" should predominate in the given case. "Casuistry" thus appeared at times to be mere "legalism" (a manipulating of "laws" or "commandments" for the sake of finding a way out of an obligation or, perhaps, of seeking to protect "law and order" by demanding more of people than is really required). Actually, the casuists were usually more profound than this, and most did not entirely deserve such an indictment. Unfortunately, however, they also considered human coitus *only* as a *bodily mechanism for conceiving a child,*[5] and *not a way of communicating love to one's spouse.*

In another typical "case" the authors taught that a husband or wife had an obligation to have sexual relations whenever his or her partner reasonably wanted them. They based this on St. Paul's teaching:

> The husband should fulfill his conjugal obligations towards his wife, and a wife hers towards her husband. A wife does not belong to herself, but to her husband; equally, a husband does not belong to himself, but to his wife. (I Cor. 7:3–4)

Practically all the casuist authors presumed that St. Paul meant literally that *a husband and wife in effect owned each other's physical reproductive system.* This quasi-ownership was achieved by the marriage *"contract"* which made over the genital powers to one's spouse so that he or she might use them as an *instrument* for having children. One author, for instance, defends a husband's right to physically force his wife to intercourse even when civil and Church law, for serious reasons, exempted her from such an obligation for a short period of time: "He does not sin . . . but simply takes what is his."[6]

The Thomistic approach which we described earlier might have raised serious questions about whether sexual union was *only* a mechanism for conceiving a child, or whether married persons truly *owned* each other's reproductive system almost as a piece of property. Unfortunately these questions were never raised. For while the casuists often applied the Thomistic approach to the *problems,* they did *not* thoroughly apply it to Biblical and church teaching or to the study of human nature where *answers* might be found. As a matter of fact, 17th century theologians like their 15th century predecessors, again almost entirely abandoned St. Thomas' approach. *This time they began to follow the ideas of René Descartes (1596–1650), who taught that the body was not a really essential part of the human person, but rather a tool used by the thinking soul.* This philoso-

27

phy simply reinforced the idea that sexual union is *only* a *mechanism* for producing a new human body.

The Popes Begin to Intervene

The inadequacy of their work notwithstanding, the writers of the *Institutiones* did a great service. Their work usually shows close contact with everyday problems, a great compassion for people's dilemmas, and a careful analysis of the facts of cases. *Without the pursuit of a more profound understanding of what God and even our own reasoning reveals to us about matters such as sexuality and marriage, however, exaggerated positions and outright errors were inevitable.* By the middle of the 17th century, a number of writers were causing serious confusion and spiritual damage. One, a Cistercian named Caramuel, wrote, for example:

> Sexual relations with another man's wife are not adultery if the husband consents to it; therefore in confession one has to mention this only as an act of fornication [that is, a sin with a single woman].[7]

Moreover, many writers were claiming that *Catholics could follow opinions such as this one simply because their authors were expert theologians*, regardless of the lack of any solid supporting arguments.[8]

Finally, Pope Alexander VII in 1665 and 1666, and Pope Innocent XI in 1679 had to condemn over 90 statements attributed to well-known theologians on moral issues. Only eight of these statements directly touched on sexual matters, it is true, but *the practice of strong papal intervention in teaching on sexual morality had begun.* It should be noted that the authors in question all affirmed the evil of adultery, fornication, homosexual acts, contraception, masturbation, and other sexual actions traditionally condemned. The problem the two Popes had to deal with was, it was alleged, the explanation and application which these authors gave to the Church's teaching.

Stability or Stagnation?

After these major papal interventions, theologians approached moral questions more cautiously. In 1750 St. Alphonsus Liguori took the papal condemnations, examined the opinions which had been debated for the previous 150 years, and commended what he considered the best opinions for use by confessors. He did not, however, enter into any profound study of the roots of moral norms.

Shortly after Alphonsus' death in 1787, the French Revolution struck and the Church's religious orders and universities were vigorously attacked in France and elsewhere. Any hope for a more profound moral theology was delayed. Napoleon's takeover of the Revolutionary forces and the wars he spawned throughout Europe only further delayed recovery of the Church's institutions for theological study.

Even when some political and social order had finally been reestablished, Catholic theologians were still influenced by *the ideas of Descartes* and by the inherited prejudice that sexual union was *only a bodily mechanism for producing a pregnancy.* This right of a husband or wife to the spouse's body was still seen as *a quasi-material right* to property and to the action for which the property was made.

In 1879 Pope Leo XIII saw that the time had come for a return to the work of Aquinas. New in-depth studies of the Scriptures and the history and writers of the early Church began. The data of modern science were more and more included. The careful analytic methods of St. Thomas began to be used. Theology was being renewed once again. This was true primarily in the area of fundamental Christian beliefs, what was called "dogmatic theology".

In the area of moral theology, however, the renewal was slower. One theologian writing in 1894 about the plight of a wife whose drunken husband wants to have sexual relations said:

> The wife is not bound to render the debt if the partner who is asking it is insane, because such a person is not capable of the use of ownership, nor does he ask with reason and in a human mode. The same is true regarding a drunken husband.[9]

While this response shows an important and growing awareness of a woman's dignity and of the limits to husband's right to conjugal relations, it also continues the older concept of quasi-material "ownership" over the body of one's spouse. Nor is there any hint here that the conjugal act is designed by God precisely to express love and esteem for one's partner.

One moral theologian, Benedict Merkelbach (1871–1942), did begin to use Aquinas' outline of moral theology according to the virtues rather than the commandments. While he also made use of some of Thomas' thought, he did not, however, basically break from the older non-Thomistic approaches. Sexual union was considered only as a God-given mechanism for having children, and not also as a sign of married love. Other great 20th century moralists such as Jerome Noldin, S. J. and Dominic Prümmer, O.P., while advancing the understanding of many moral issues, nonetheless left unasked questions which had been waiting a long time.

Sexual Union as an Expression of Conjugal Love[10]

In 1928, Dietrich von Hildebrand attracted considerable attention by insisting again, with some other authors, that the conjugal act is meant to express conjugal love, and that, without love, the mere physical aspect of sexual union is immoral. In 1935 Herbert Doms marshaled an impressive array of scholarly arguments to support the same view. Bernard Häring indicated at least some agreement with it in 1959, and Joseph Fuchs, in 1960, expressed total agreement. The leading American moralists, John Ford and Gerard Kelly, wrote in 1963:

> These acts . . . are not merely appropriate expressions of love, but they are *necessarily* expressions of love. That is, they are so typically acts of love that one cannot imagine an obligation to them which does not presuppose them to be acts of the virtue of love.[11]

Thus on the eve of the Second Vatican Council a number of authors had come a long way from the view that the conjugal act is purely a mechanism for procreation or an exercise of ownership over another person's body. *These new authors were saying that, within marriage, the physical act is designed by God always to be a sign of love.* At the same time, *against the growing contraception movement,* all of these authors were affirming that this act is of necessity *the very same act by which children can be conceived* if God wills at that point to create a new human being.

Official Teaching Faces Contemporary Issues

As this new development began to take hold among theologians from 1880 to 1960 the Popes and the Bishops repeatedly defended married love against the growing acceptance of divorce. The same was true regarding the contraception issue, where *the reaction against the growing birth control movement represented a world-wide Catholic position.* As one proponent of abandoning this position was later to write:

The instructions from Rome from 1816 to 1930 had interacted with the acts of the national hierarchies. It would be a mistake, I believe, to see the national statements against contraception as dictated from Rome, or the Roman interventions as brought about by national demands. A common tradition and theological training, supervised from Rome, suffices to explain the harmony of action. *Casti Connubii* was the high-water mark. It guided action for the next thirty-four years.[12]

Casti Connubii was the encyclical letter of Pope Pius XI in 1930. It was the first letter on sexual morality written by a pope to the worldwide Church. Two of its more important passages refer to *the place of love in marriage* and to the essential relation the conjugal act has to *the procreation of children.*

> *(This unity in marriage excludes sexual relations with anyone but one's spouse.) This kind of unity is made much easier and happier and more ennobling, and will flourish from another source which is most outstanding, namely, conjugal love, which pervades all the obligations of conjugal life and in Christian marriage holds, indeed, a kind of primacy.*[13]

While not adopting the position of the theologians who saw sexual union as the central act for expressing conjugal love, Pius XI here in no way condemns their position, and even offers some encouragement for it.

Regarding the relation of sexual union to procreation, the Pope writes

> *But as a matter of fact there is no reason, not even a most serious one, which can bring it about that what is intrinsically against nature can become consonant with nature and a good act. Since, however, by its very nature the conjugal act is destined for the begetting of children, those who, in making use of it, by their own intervention deprive it of this natural force and power act against nature and do something impure and intrinsically immoral.*[14]

Pius XII (1939–1958), in his many discourses to medical professionals, applied previous official teaching in a more detailed way. The following brief summaries of official teaching regarding contraception and other issues which could touch more directly on medical ethics are based on these discourses of Pius XII. For each of the following topics it will be important to note a) what the Church's teaching said; b) what reasons it gave, if any; and c) what the Church did not say.[15]

1) *Artificial Contraception*

a) *What Church teaching said.* One may not freely choose sexual union and then change its fundamental physiological structure in order to avoid a pregnancy. Thus all actions are ruled out by which a man pursues sexual action, but deliberately releases his seed elsewhere than into his wife's vagina, either by withdrawal, by using a condom, or by any other change in the structure of the sexual act. The same is true of a wife who willingly enters into sexual union, but then rejects her husband's semen by some barrier, such as a diaphragm, a spermicide or a douche.

b) *Reasons given for the teaching.* Such changes in the structure of the sexual act are said simply to be "against nature" because the sexual union is "destined for begetting children." Whether God intends this begetting of children to be the direct result of physical union, or whether He intends this begetting to take place only when the physical union is an expression of genuine mutual love is a question not raised.

c) *What Church teaching did not say.* Official teachings do not discuss the use of artificial means of avoiding pregnancy for wives who, in a given instance, have a right to refrain from sexual actions, but are truly forced into them by abusive husbands.

2) *Sterilization*

a) *What Church teaching said.* It is wrong to destroy or deactivate the generative powers of the human body unless the overall good of the person cannot be provided for in any other way. Thus, governmental sterilization programs, such as the Nazi ones in the 1930's, to provide for the genetic "improvement" of the race are specifically condemned. Moreover, couples must at times meet personal and family problems such as health and finances by a free and responsible decision to curtail or, in rare cases, to avoid sexual actions rather than to mutilate the body of one or both partners by surgery, drugs, or any other means.

b) *Reason given for the teaching.* The body in all its aspects is a gift of God, Who has with loving care provided for its basic structure and in a special way its sexual structure. Man's right to change that structure is limited to cases where he has no other way of solving a serious threat to his health or personal dignity.

When, for instance, a person can freely choose to refrain from sexual actions rather than seek sterilization, he or she must do so.

c) *What Church teaching did not say.* A dispute arose among theologians in 1960 as to whether sterilization could be used, at least as a last resort, to save women threatened by rape from being impregnated. Official teaching did not publicly favor one side or the other.

3) *Natural Family Planning*

a) *What Church teaching said.* Using only the infertile periods of a woman's ovulation cycle for sexual union is justified if the couple has serious reasons for avoiding a pregnancy. The use of the infertile periods by a couple as an expression of an unwillingness to accept their vocation to give life would be wrong.

b) *Reasons given for the teaching.* The obligation of couples to actually conceive children is real but limited.

c) *What Church teaching did not say.* Official teaching does not require that Catholics "get permission" in Confession to use the infertile periods.

4) *Masturbation*

a) *What Church teaching said.* Masturbation cannot be justified for therapeutic reasons, such as relieving tension, or for seminal analysis or neurological diagnosis, for artificial insemination, or for research purposes.

b) *Reasons given for the teaching.* Masturbation is contrary to man's sexual nature, which requires that the orgasmic release be in every instance at the service of bringing children into the world and taking care of them.

c) *What Church teaching did not say.* Official teaching does not discuss the use of *part* of the semen released in a conjugal act for diagnosis or research, nor the obtaining of a semen specimen through nonorgasmic acts such as prostate massage.

5) *Artificial Insemination and In Vitro Fertilization*

a) *What Church teaching said.* Even where semen can be obtained through non-orgasmic means it may not then be injected into a wife's reproductive tract by artificial means in order to achieve a pregnancy.

b) *Reasons given for the teaching.* The conjugal act in its obvious natural structure is an expression of the love between husband and wife. God wills children to be conceived only out of this highly personal expression of love.

c) *What Church teaching did not say.* The teaching does not condemn medical techniques which aid the structure of the conjugal act in achieving a pregnancy, but leave that structure basically as God has made it. Thus techniques which aid or sustain erection, or seek to transfer the already deposited semen further into wife's reproductive tract are not ruled out.

6) *Homosexuality. Treatment of Rape Victims, and Sex Therapy for Impotency and Frigidity*
These issues had not surfaced in a controversial way among Catholic theologian before the Second Vatican Council. Official teaching, then, without comment, allowed the common teaching of theologians on these issues to stand as a safe guide.

Conclusion

The period from roughly the discovery of America to the Second Vatican Council showed that the Church was stable in its fundamental convictions about what sexual life must mean for the human being as a person and as a Christian. At the same time, her theologians and her bishops expected and achieved a deepening of understanding of human sexuality. That deepening was to prove necessary and invaluable for facing newly rising challenges to, and even attacks on, traditional moral attitudes. It would also prepare the way for the collegial work of the Bishops in the Second Vatican Council (1962–1965).

Discussion Questions

1. Why did the highest levels of Church authority for many centuries see little reason to speak out about sexual morality?
2. Did St. Thomas believe that we could truly understand anything fundamental about ourselves as persons? What three sources of knowledge about human beings did he seek carefully to analyze?
3. What philosophers began to undo his work? How did they pave the way for the Protestant movement in the 16th century?
4. Why did Catholic moralists in the 16th century not develop a deep analysis and defense of Catholic moral tradition?
5. Name two inadequate ideas which moralists from the 16th to the 20th century had regarding sexual intercourse.
6. Why did Popes Alexander VII and Innocent XI begin to speak out on moral issues?

7. When did prominent theologians in modern times begin to explore the fact that the sexual act is a sign of love? Did these authors therefore accept contraception?

8. In the teachings of the Church summarized at the end of this chapter, what indications are there that sexual union is designed by God to be a sign of love?

Notes

1. Peter Damian, *The Book of Gamorrah*, trans. Pierre J. Payer, (Waterloo, Ontario, Wilfred Laurier Press, 1982) pp. 95–97. See also *The Church Teaches* (St. Louis, Herder, 1964), n. 335 for the Fourth Lateran Council's defense of marriage, and n. 854 for its indissolubility.

2. See Parmisano above in Chapter Two, footnote 6.

3. For a profile of Catholic theology in the 15th and 16th century, see James Weisheipl, "Thomism," in the *New Catholic Encyclopedia*, hereafter NCE, (New York, McGraw-Hill, 1967), Vol. 14, pp. 132–135.

4. Edward Hamel, "Casuistry" in NCE above, Vol. 3, pp. 195–197.

5. Charles Curran, *The Prevention of Pregnancy After Rape* (Rome, The Gregorian University, 1960).

6. Francisus Lopez de Texeda, *Controversiae Theologiae Moralis*, 1646, quoted in Edward Bayer, *Rape Within Marriage: A Moral Analysis Delayed*, (Lanliam, M.D., 1985: University Press of America), p. 19–20.

7. Henricus Denzinger et Adolfus Schönmetzer, S.J., *Enchiridion Symbolorum*, editio XXXVI emendata, (Romae, Herder, 1976), n. 2150 with its footnote.

8. F. J. Connell, "Laxism," in NCE above, Vol. 8, p. 573.

9. Dominic Palmieri in his 1894 revision of Anthony Ballerini's work, cited and quoted in Bayer, above, pp. 50–52.

10. Noonan, *op. cit.*, pp. 491–504.

11. John Ford and Gerard Kelly, *Contemporary Moral Theology*, (Westminster, Newman, 1964), Vol. II, p. 117.

12. Noonan, above, pp. 431–432.

13. Denzinger-Schönmetzer, above, 3707.

14. See the collection of papal teachings in *The Human Body* (Boston, Daughters of St. Paul, 1979) nn. 8–11.

15. *Ibid.*, nn. 59, 174–179, 268, 280, 496, 505.

Preview of Chapter Four

● New medical technology makes it possible to fundamentally redesign human sexual relations which God has created.

● Wars, economic crisis, consumerism, and organized socio-political movements create a discontent towards traditional sexual morality.

● Intellectual elites hand on the doubts of philosophers prior to the 20th century about our capacity to know that any specific kind of action is wrong without exception. The only moral norm is to produce the most pleasurable earthly life possible.

● Protestant churches generally abandon their traditional stance against artificial contraception, and move toward Situation Ethics.

● Doubts grow in certain Catholic circles regarding Church teaching about contraception and fundamentals of morality.

CHAPTER 4

Twentieth Century Challenges to Traditional Sexual Morality

In Chapter 3 we saw that the Catholic Church has taken an official position on a number of moral questions, including some that touch upon human sexuality. In doing this the Church was speaking to real flesh and blood persons faced with the opportunities and the problems of everyday life, and subjected to many outside influences. *Friends and neighbors, governments and schools, mass media, the entertainment industry, the economy, and the science of the 20th century, all challenged individuals and couples whose moral dilemmas the Church was addressing.*

What have these 20th century challenges been like? And how did it feel to be subjected to them in the period prior to the opening of the Second Vatican Council in 1963?

Some of these challenges have been very *visible* and *obvious;* others, in contrast have been immensely influential in a *very subtle* way. In the present chapter we shall examine both types.

Technological Challenges

Dr. Robert Frederickson, a leading American physician and medical researcher, writing shortly after President Reagan took office, described the changes in the field of medicine alone in the 20th century as nothing less than a revolution:

> Never has there been a comparable period of growth in the knowledge of living things. *The current revolution in the life sciences is not a simple, linear projection of the growth curve in knowledge for the past century. A striking perturbation of that growth has occurred, amounting to a geometric progression of available information.* Achievements of research in chemistry, physics, and many allied disciplines during this same period have led to new technologies contributing to a flood of discovery in biochemistry, physiology, and medicine. Our ignorance is still vast, but we are on the threshold of some unusual transformations in health practices, agriculture, and industry.[1]

The *amount of growth* in biological knowledge and in *its technological application,* then, can rightly be termed *disturbing,* at least in the sense that *no one individual can absorb it all.* Nor is the human *community* at all confident that it can *channel all of this "knowledge explosion" in a healthy direction, or even keep it from doing a great deal of harm.* And what is true here regarding the strictly biological sciences is true also regarding other sciences such as chemistry and physics. Witness our great concern over chemical pollution and, even more, over nuclear disasters.

The individual inside or outside marriage is affected by all this and, if he or she is a responsible person, is concerned. Many would say that, if people have any sense, they are even worried.

Advances in the biological sciences during this century included immense advances in life-saving techniques and medicines. As a result, *life expectancy has risen dramatically in many parts of the world.* At the same time, world population figures have risen rapidly and a "population explosion" is of real concern to many. Medical advances may also have served to lower inhibitions about sexual promiscuity, since *many people, correctly or not began no longer to fear the ravages of venereal disease.* Safer and more effective surgical techniques have also contributed to lessening the fear of abortions, surgical sterilizations, and transsexual operations. The development of the new anovulant drugs and intrauterine devices, as well as the improving of condoms and pessaries already in use at the turn of the century,[2] have left millions with *the impression that contraceptive practices are at last safe and sound,* an impression which, as we note in Chapter 9, may be open to question. One segment after another of the medical community wrote off as "antiquated" traditional rejections of masturbation as a sub-human act, and even advocated it for "release of tension" or even for "mental health". The morality of masturbation for the collection of semen for diagnostic or research purposes was taken for granted in medical circles outside the influence of the Catholic Church. Homosexual acts came to be treated more and more in the same way. Finally new techniques for producing a pregnancy without normal sexual intercourse were invented.

The rapid development of these and other aspects of the biological sciences, then, could not fail to test the individuals and the couples who had to deal with both the offerings and the offal of life in the 20th century.

Sociological Challenges

The good and bad aspects of 20th century life, often inextricably intertwined, show themselves in major patterns of life today. Indeed these patterns are so familiar that *it is often difficult to appreciate how dramatic were the sociological changes which brought them into being.*

The effect of World War I (1914–1918) and World War II (1939–1944) in preparing these changes and the challenges they brought to traditional morality cannot be entirely discounted. The agonies and atrocities of war can produce traumas which unsettle even the healthiest and deepest of human convictions. Since these two wars were *worldwide* in scope, they took thousands of young men who otherwise might never have left home to distant parts of the world. There was more than a modicum of wisdom in the popular World War I song: "How you gonna' keep 'em down on the farm/After they've seen Par-èe?" It was not the farm that was so immediately at stake however; it was *a man's whole previous vision of life.* World War II took America's youth to even more distant shores, with their new and different outlooks on life. *Many returned more committed than ever to traditional moral values; many did not.*

After World War I, "the roaring 20's" laid bare the moral disorientation of millions, often epitomized by celebrities from the society and entertainment worlds as they flaunted their break with moral tradition. *While many ordinary citizens resisted their examples, many others followed.*

In 1900 there were 7 divorces for every 100 persons; by 1925 the rate had doubled.³ Though contraceptives were widely used, both venereal disease and abortions increased. The "crash" of the economy in 1929 also caused the crash of many dreams, and *a desperation which drove many couples to artificial contraception.*

The same industrial-economic structure which lay almost paralyzed in the Great Depression slowly rose from its collapse only to create yet more challenges to sexual morality. Aside from recurrent "recessions," the developing patterns of business life often also demanded an increased willingness of workers to move from one part of the nation to another. This was especially true if a man hoped to "go up in the company." This requirement, in turn, weakened the "extended family" pattern, that is, the "nuclear" family of husband, wife and children was no longer in frequent personal contact with the children's grandparents, aunts, uncles, and cousins. *Without the example, encouragement, and aid of the extended family it was for many couples extremely difficult to maintain the ideals of an older generation.*

The same economic developments also began to demand that more women should work outside the home. This was often an unavoidable necessity. *More frequently, however, it was the result of an ever increasing desire for material goods.* This desire was constantly whetted by business interests through ever more sophisticated mass media campaigns.

The mass-media in the 20th century not only appealed to the materialism to which human beings are so prone, but also served to offer direct challenges to traditional attitudes towards sexuality. As is well known, the rising motion picture industry showed divorce both on and off the silver screen. The marital misadventures and other sexual misadventures, as well as drug, alcohol abuse and other personal problems of many of its leading personages were—and still are—world famous. Television, radio, and popular journals treated their audiences to more and more "neutral" discussions of divorce and birth control. Magazines of the *Playboy* type began to appear in the early 1960's. They sold sexual pursuits separated from marital commitment, as well as the consumption of luxury items as a necessary part of the healthy male's life. "Humor" in the form of cartoons belittled traditional moral sensitivities by portraying even sexual acts with animals and children as somehow "amusing". *A constant barrage of this type of philosophy could not fail to insinuate doubts about the worth of sexual self-control and the simple joys of family life.*

The "new morality" has been focused more and more clearly throughout the 20th century in *organized* movements which frequently promoted one or more challenges to traditional morality.⁴ Though protagonists of artificial contraception had spoken out occasionally as early as 1797, it was only in 1900 in Paris that the First International Congress on Birth Control was held. Other such Congresses followed in 1905, 1910, 1911 and 1922. In 1925 the sixth one was held in New York City. In 1927 a headquarters for the movement was set up in Geneva, Switzerland. The American Margaret Sanger organized a national society to promote birth control in the United States in 1913, and established clinics here and in other countries.

By 1935 several hundred types of chemical and mechanical contraceptives were on the market. All the most prestigious medical schools instructed their students in their use.[5] With the singular exception of the Catholic Church, almost all western religious bodies abandoned their traditional opposition to artificial contraception. Many became advocates of it. By 1960, as the Second Vatican Council opened, the success of the birth control movement had begun an erosion of certitude in issues of sexual morality. *The full implications of this erosion however, would appear only after that Council had ended.*

The abortion movement did not make quite the same progress. Nonetheless some elite groups did begin to press for more permissive laws in 1961, and for this purpose the American Law Institute drafted a model law which state legislatures might follow. In 1962 Colorado's legislature did precisely that.[6] A new challenge to traditional morality thus surfaced. It was one to which the Second Vatican Council, just opening, would have to speak.

Prior to the Second Vatican Council, then, the great advance in medical science, the disruptions of two world wars and of the Great Depression, and the rise of certain militant and organized movements *led many to wonder if the norms of sexual morality previously taken for granted were valid any longer.*

The Subtle Challenges of the Thinkers

Twentieth-century developments in the life sciences and the changes in society which have been described thus far were obvious to the average citizen who read the newspaper. *Other influences* on people were *just as real,* though perhaps *not so obvious.* These were the influences of *philosophers, that is, the thinkers who in every century attempt to state,* however feebly, *the most basic truths about the human race.* These statements of basic truths inevitably shape not only our picture of what human beings are, but also *how they should live.*

When this country was founded, many of its leading citizens were committed to a philosophic approach called *naturalism.* They believed that the powers of *natural human intelligence alone* enabled human beings

41

to know *all that is necessary* about *themselves* and *how they should live ethically.* In the final analysis, they thought, the human person did not need anything *revealed* to him by God regarding religious or moral life. Moreover, their emphasis on what unaided human reason could discover on its own led also to a great emphasis on the sciences then emerging with new accuracy in the eighteenth century, and on the great promise these sciences offered when applied to human problems. Because leading figures of the eighteenth century looked so expectantly to the *light* which human reason could throw on human ethical and scientific questions, their program for humanity came to be known as *The Enlightenment.*

The use of nothing but the natural power of human reasoning, however, wound up leaving many people with perplexing doubts. Leaders of the Enlightenment—usually members of the more educated aristocracy—were split among themselves as to whether God, once He had created the universe, has continued to intervene in its history—or even whether a "God" exists at all who cares one way or another about how we live. Others professed simply not to know the answers to these questions,—a position which came to known as *agnosticism* (from the Greek *"a"*—"no", and *"gnosis"*—"knowledge").

Many of these naturalist aristocrats imbued with the ideals of the Enlightenment among the founders of the new United States of America. All of them well-educated aristocrats who feared, however, that, among *ordinary* citizens, this naturalistic approach of theirs would lead to a total breakdown of morality. And so, whatever the moral quality, or sometimes lack of it, of their own personal lives, they spoke and wrote publicly in favor of traditional moral norms in very much the same sense in which the Catholic and other Christian churches upheld them. They were, in a certain sense, living off the Christian past of their ancestors.

One leading German naturalist philosopher, Immanuel Kant (1724–1804), was raised a devout Lutheran, but by the end of his life had abandoned much of his Christian faith.[9] He did not depart, however, from traditional Christian moral norms, though he maintained that the human conscience, unaided by any revelation, could discover these norms. Nonetheless, later philosophic naturalists moved farther and farther from them.

Nonetheless, these same philosophic naturalists continued to try to establish by human reason alone *some* kind of "ultimate goals" worthy of human beings. Their efforts since the days of Kant have filtered down into ways of thinking even among people of our century, especially in Europe and the nations of North and South America. This is true particularly of the following four approaches to ethics and various versions and combinations of them.

1) *Pleasure-centered utilitarianism.*

In England, Jeremy Bentham (1748–1832) preached an ego-centered hedonism which, for its foundation, asked only one question: "Will the act I am now considering doing produce the greatest amount of pleasure and eliminate the greatest amount of pain for the greatest possible number of persons affected by my act?"[10] Thus the usefulness or utility of an act in producing *the one thing important to produce*—for Bentham, it was *pleasure*—was the only thing that mattered ultimately. Bentham's approach came to be known as *utilitarianism.* It is interesting to note that Bentham was one of the first to advocate contraceptive "sponges" to limit the number of poor people and thus lower taxes needed for their support.

2) *Utilitarianism centered on other ultimate goals than pleasure.*

Later naturalist philosophers quickly rejected Bentham's maximizing of pleasure as the ultimate moral norm, but held out other goods as morally "the ultimate goal" to be aimed at. A few examples of the various "ultimate goals" they proposed were:

> development of each individual's total personality by his or her own creative effort, and the abolition of all laws—or even mere societal disapproval—which would in any way discourage this (J. S. Mill);

> freedom to express human passions, and the establishment of a world entirely of small, highly individualistic self-sufficient communities without any government over them (C. Fourier);

> openness to a total abandonment of all traditional moral norms and patterns for living (P. Prouhdon); and

> a perfect society needing no government because all members are totally equal in material goods (K. Marx).

People who bought into these different versions of "the ultimate goal" also easily applied to these goals the *utilitarianism* which Bentham previously had applied to pleasure: any means to achieve "the ultimate goal" is morally acceptable. Once accepted, this maxim would inevitably be applied to sexual activity—and was. It could be morally justified, this kind of utilitarianism held, for people to depart totally from the normal structure and meaning of sexual orgasm in the conjugal act. All that is ethically necessary to justify such a change is that it significantly contribute to achieving whatever one has identified as life's "ultimate goal".

3) *Purely statistical sociology.*

The Frenchman, Auguste Compte (1798–1857), wanted a purely *statistical study* of how human beings actually live.[11] He did not recognize any ethical norm for judging that way of living nor for asking whether it needed to be changed in light of any teachings from God or even any profound rational questions.

Once accepted, Compte's approach led people easily to be satisfied with doing whatever the majority in society accepted as allowable. If most people—or even a significant number—accepted sexual practices which departed from the traditional Christian or even rational norm, the temptation was to presume that these practices were not to be questioned.

4) *The Human will as source of order.*

Friedrich Nietzsche (1844–1900), one of a number of atheist philosophers, urged the willful smashing of all designs that allegedly came from a "God".[12] For Nietzsche, there was no hope of *discovering* a "right" or "wrong". Instead, it was up to a superior portion of the human race intelligently to *plan out* what should be "right" and "wrong", and then to impose that plan upon other human beings,—to bring the world "new order".

It should be noted here that, though the German Nazi movement picked up this idea, the Nazis carried it in some instances beyond anything which Nietzsche would have approved. They did not hesitate, for instance, to apply it:

1) to official programs promoting extra-marital pregnancies which would supply more "pure aryan" children for the building up of the Third Reich; or
2) to eliminating for "eugenically less desirable" elements in the German population (e.g., Jews and the mentally or physically below average), or among conquered nations (e.g., certain groups among the Poles) by sterilization—or, if necessary, extermination.

Utilitarianism, applied to the above mentioned and other "ultimate goals", was handed on to Americans largely through the influence of

44

John Dewey (1859–1952) who influenced thousands of aspiring teachers through his books and the philosophy courses he taught for 35 years at the Teachers' College of Columbia University.[13] These teachers in turn formed thousands of other teachers at the state level, and thus eventually affected millions of children in public and even private schools. Dewey's influence on American law through his friend and admirer, Supreme Court Justice Oliver Wendell Holmes, is generally admitted. Both became identified with the philosophy that a judge should if necessary ignore the original meaning of previously passed laws and even of the Constitution itself, and render decisions contrary to that meaning. This new legislation by the court should be guided by *utilitarian* principles: Will the judge's ruling produce more progress than problems for society as a whole?

As we have seen, in many people's thinking, the "progress" which the law should produce, means simply "pleasure". When the law affects access to sexual pleasure, the best law then would be that which provides or at least safeguards the maximum amount of sexual pleasure for the maximum number of persons affected by that law. But, as those who rejected Bentham's pleasure-utilitarianism noted, this mentality simply ignores questions which have to be answered:

Is the *physical* pleasure or good of human beings the *only* factor to be considered in making ethical decisions? *Or is there another kind of pleasure?* Is there pleasure in the simple *discovery* of the *wise plans and loving intentions* of another person? Is there *another Person Who is above and beyond all human life, yet deeply present and involved* in the world and the human persons He has created? Is there a kind of *spiritual* pleasure which man experiences when he recognizes that his body—with its sexuality— is not just an accident, but *a gift* lovingly thought out and provided by his Maker? Is man made to experience this deep pleasure of intellect and will in seeing and embracing the plan which *God* has wrought? *Can the human being truly be happy without doing this?*

As we have seen also, other thinkers would identify the "progress" which law is supposed to produce with the individual's development, or with a society of totally equal distribution of wealth, or one where constant technological and organizational progress is being made, etc. Such a mentality would not be closed at all to laws and pressures promoting sterilization, or sexual acts outside marriage (by heterosexual or homosexual persons, whether alone or with others), or surrogate parenting, or forming animal-human hybrids. These would not be wrong, nor would any other departures from what both the Christian and even most rational moral tradition has held to be the only humanly worthwhile expression of human sexuality: the conjugal act. Such departures from either the physiological structure or the human meaning of this

45

act could be justified, these utilitarians would hold, for purposes of scientific research, or for medical and other technology, or for solving social problems of feeding or housing people, or for military and national security reasons, etc. Human beings are morally free to change their sexuality as they choose as long as the change is "useful".

But again, like the pleasure-utilitarianism of Bentham, this mentality also leaves certain questions unanswered, but this time about *human cleverness.* Can the human race be truly satisfied as individuals or as a society if it cannot recognize that more than *human technological and organizational cleverness* governs life? When does such cleverness come to the point of violating, rather than serving, human persons? How can we know when we have reached this destructive point, if we do not have sure knowledge about at least some basic, ultimate realities about our human selves—including our sexuality? Is there some design to our sexuality which is *not* of our making, and which must be respected if we are to survive as *authentically* human sexual persons? And are there perhaps even *deeper* meanings to our sexuality than even the finest human mind can uncover,—meanings which come from and lead to eternity,—meanings which our Maker alone can reveal to us?

Though many of the influential thinkers of the 20th century would not treat these questions seriously, *the questions did not go away.* Great numbers of people, meanwhile, were faced with the national and international upheavals described in the first part of this chapter. Developments in the biological sciences offered relatively easy solutions to one of their main problems, the control of family size. Under these circumstances, the subtle pull of the philosophies current among the intellectually elite was felt and, for better or for worse, the erosion of a moral tradition had begun.

Theological Challenges

Far more influential than the philosophers for the average American were the churches. The history of their stance on issues of sexuality in the 20th century reveals still further challenges to fundamentals of traditional moral teaching.

Protestantism in the 19th and 20th centuries is marked by two seemingly contradictory movements, namely liberalism and literalism.[14] Prior to 1900, the mainline churches were deeply affected by the scientific studies of the origins and meanings of the Biblical texts. *These studies began to create a scepticism among both clergy and laity as to the applicability of moral norms as they are found in the Scriptures.* At the same time, those who were most affected by this scepticism were attracted more and more to what came to be known as "The Social Gospel," the moral obligation to improve the living conditions of the more disadvantaged in our society. Though doctrinal themes basic to Christianity continued to be preached, some of them were muted, denied, or at least given a new interpretation which many Protestants found difficult to recognize as the faith of their fathers.

As a result, other Protestants, at times whole churches of them, took a strongly conservative turn toward literalism. This meant a strong emphasis on the face value of any passage in the Bible, without relying on modern sciences or theories to correct possible previous misunderstandings by Christian scholars as to what the original writers intended to present as the word of God Himself. For instance, had most Christians been inaccurate in presuming that the biblical books intend to insist that the world was created in only six days? Or was this simply a commonplace description three thousand years ago which the biblical writers picked up in order to say what really counted: that one and only God was responsible for the existence of all the world—regardless of the exact process or timetable He used? Could scientific and historical help answer these questions? No, said the fundamentalists: the centuries-old presumption that creation was a six day process was correct. *The same conservative spirit insisted also on an adherence to and promotion of moral traditions peculiar to American Protestantism.*

In the United States, this adherence showed itself in the largely Protestant-backed passage in 1914 of the 18th Constitutional Amendment, which attempted practically to abolish all use of alcoholic drinks from the American scene.[15] *When the same amendment was repealed in 1933, much of the moral influence of the more popular, conservative branch of Protestantism suffered a great loss.*

The confusion among Protestants as to how to handle pressing social problems soon caused a major change in one area of sexual morality, artificial contraception.[16] An outstanding example was the Protestant Episcopal Church. Two worldwide meetings of Anglican (Episcopalian) bishops, at Lambeth, England in 1908 and 1920, had reiterated the traditional Protestant condemnations of artificial contraception. In 1925 the American Episcopalian bishops followed their lead and did the same. By 1930, however, the Lambeth meeting had completely reversed its position, and the Episcopal Church in the United States followed suit.

An attempt was made, especially in Europe after World War II, to justify this and other changes in Protestant moral teachings. The attempt took the form of *Situation Ethics,* which recognized the sinfulness of many decisions to which the situations of life force us, but insisted that the mercy of God would somehow make those sinful decisions right. In the United States, the Episcopalian theologian Joseph Fletcher defended Situation

Ethics against many Protestant critics and insisted that *it was basically no different than the teaching most of them already espoused.*[17] It was simply an attempt to blend *utilitarianism* with *classical Protestant doctrine.*

The Catholic Church not only did not reverse her teaching on contraception, but strongly affirmed that position. Many theologians, however, began to recognize that they had not succeeded well up to that time in showing how the sexual act was, in God's plan, an expression of the couple's love. This deficiency in theologians' work made it difficult to explain the Church's teaching or to defend it adequately.

Around the time that the Second Vatican Council opened, however, a growing number of clergy and laity were *beginning to doubt the teaching itself.* Some began to formulate explanations as to how the teaching could be reversed without contradicting basic Catholic doctrine. Eventually they moved to theories claiming that the Church could not rule out *situations* which would allow a person *licitly* to choose *contraceptive or other sexual actions traditionally condemned in her teaching.*[18]

The Second Vatican Council: Challenged and Challenging

As the Council opened in 1963, the full implications of the wide acceptance of artificial contraception and of Situation Ethics in its various versions had not yet surfaced. *It was only after the Council that Catholic theologians favoring a "Catholic version* these two positions began to follow out the logic of Protestants who championed them.* Within a few years, and especially after 1968 when Pope Paul VI reiterated the Church's condemnation of artificial contraception, Catholics who rejected that condemnation were arguing that *there could be situations* in which one would be *justified in pursuing homosexual, masturbatory, pre-marital, and extra-marital sexual actions as somehow compatible with the Christian life.* The Church and her people had been challenged, but both during and after the Council they were to do some challenging of their own.

Discussion Questions

1. In what way have medical advances made departures from traditional sexual morality easier?
2. How has American economic life since the Great Depression of 1929 tended to break down the traditional pattern of family life?
3. Did the 18th century emphasis on total reliance on human reason produce a widespread certitude in moral matters?

4. What is utilitarianism? How did it eventually affect American religious thinkers?
5. What happened to Protestant moral teaching after World War I?
6. Did all Catholics reject positions resembling Protestant Situation Ethics?

Notes

1. Donald S. Frederickson, M.D., "Biomedical Research in the 1980's," *The New England Journal of Medicine*, February 26, 1981, p. 509.

2. John Noonan, *Contraception: A History of Its Treatment by the Catholic Theologians and Canonists*. (Cambridge, Belknap, 1965), pp. 491–504, 347–350, 394, 408, 460–461.

3. W. F. Kenkle, "Divorce" in *New Catholic Encyclopedia*, hereafter NCE, (New York, McGraw-Hill, 1967), Vol. 4, p. 929.

4. Noonan, *loc. cit.*

5. *Ibid.*, pp. 407–409.

6. John Noonan, *A Private Choice*, (New York, Macmillan, 1979) pp. 22–23, 34, 35, 53, 58.

7. G. J. Dalcourt, "Ethics, Rise of," in NCE, Vol. 5, 575–577.

8. Noonan, *Contraception, op. cit.*, pp. 409 and pp. 490–491.

9. Dalcourt, *op. cit.*, p. 576.

10. R. I. Cunningham, "Bentham, Jeremy," in NCE, Vol. 2, p. 314. Cf. also Noonan, *op. cit.*, pp. 392–393.

11. R. A. Nisbet, "Compte, Auguste," in NCE. Vol. 4, pp. 100–101.

12. K. F. Reinhardt, "Nietzsche, Friedrich," in NCE, pp. 463–464.

13. J. P. Dougherty, "Dewey, John," in NCE. Vol. 4, pp. 835–836.

14. G. H. Tavard, "Protestantism," in NCE. Vol. 11, p. 898; and A. Dulles, "Fundamentalism," *ibid.*, Vol. 6, pp. 223–224.

15. P. Kibre, "Temperance Movements," in NCE. Vol. 13, pp. 990–991.

16. Noonan, *loc. cit.*

17. Joseph Fletcher, *Storm over Ethics* (United Church Press, 1967), pp. 151–152.

18. *Ibid.* pp. 153–155 and pp. 171–172.

Preview of
Chapter Five

● The document on "The Church in the Modern World" of the Second Vatican Council sees the marital act in a personalist context in which spouses express what God made them to be as individuals and to be for each other in their sexual activity.

● The Council emphasized that the conjugal act, more than being merely a bodily mechanism for procreation, is a sign which speaks both of the mutual love of spouses and the procreational nature of that love.

● The controversy within the Papal Commission on Population, the Family, and Births did not focus on the integrist personalism which was emerging. This position holds that accepting one's sexual nature is a kind of worship of God and taking apart the sexual act is offensive to Him.

● Pope Paul VI in his encyclical, *Humanae Vitae*, concentrates on marital acts as God-given signs of the relationship between husband and wife. He emphasizes that the act must be a genuine, unaltered, and complete expression of conjugal love and rejects contraception.

● In 1981 Pope John Paul II in *Familiaris Consortio* (On the Family) rejects separatist personalism and accepts integrist personalism.

CHAPTER 5

Vatican II and Subsequent Church Teaching

God has chosen to make the human race "in His image and likeness" (Gen. 1:27) precisely by wanting individuals to be male or female. The Church, as was seen in Chapter Three, has striven down through the ages to uncover more and more completely the richness of this divine decision.

Christians daily face the challenge of living as true images of God in every aspect of their lives, including their sexuality. As Chapter 4 showed, however, *there are challenges special to the present time which call forth new questions and demand deeper answers about the human sexuality which God has created,* as well as about all other aspects of a truly Catholic, Christian, and human life.

Pope John XXIII during his few years (1958–1963) of service "in the place of Peter" was aware of what Catholics, especially theologians, had already been doing to at least begin to face the challenges of the twentieth century. He was convinced also, however, that the time had come for those who, as bishops, bear the primary pastoral responsibility in the Church to come together in what was to be called the Second Vatican Council.

Almost a year and a half before the Council, however, on May 15, 1961, he himself spoke to one issue of sexual morality in *Mater et Magistra* (The Church, Mother and Teacher). For in touching on the need for population control, Pope John wrote:

> Because the life of man is passed on to other men deliberately and knowingly, it therefore follows that this should be done in accord with the most sacred, permanent, inviolate prescriptions of God. Everyone without exception is bound to recognize and observe these laws. Wherefore, in this matter, no one is permitted to use methods and procedures which may indeed be permissible to control the life of animals and plants.[1]

While treating of many other challenges to the Church's life in today's world, the Council would have to affirm once again and plumb to greater depths than ever these "most sacred, permanent, and inviolate prescriptions of God" for the transmission of human life.

In another encyclical, Pope John also criticized the age-old presumption that women were in any sense mere instruments for the carrying out of men's plans:

> Far from being content with a purely passive role or allowing themselves to be regarded as a kind of instrument, women are demanding both in domestic and in public life the rights and duties which belong to them as human persons.[2]

While not speaking explicitly to sexual issues, this emphatic statement could not leave unshaken certain attitudes towards sexuality.

The Second Vatican Council, 1963–1965

One document more than any other produced by the 2400 bishops at the Second Vatican Council speaks to issues of sexuality and marriage: *Gaudium et Spes*, the "Pastoral Constitution on the Church in the Modern World." Moreover, in no other issues are both the complex problems of the modern world and the work of theologians prior to the

Council more in evidence. *For both the problems and the theology made it obvious to the bishops that the conjugal act could no longer be treated as a totally physiological act. Nor could it be treated as an act with the single purpose of producing a pregnancy.* It had to be seen rather as a *personalist act,* that is, an act by which a *person* expressed *what God had made him or her to be in his or her sexuality,* and *what He had made two persons to be in their married love for each other.*

Hindsight now makes it obvious, however, that, as the Council progressed, *two incompatible versions* surfaced among theologians as to *what this personalist approach really meant.* We might call one view *integrist* personalism. "Integrist" comes from the Latin word *"integer"* which means "entire." Integrist theologians immediately prior to the Council had seen the obvious physical form of the conjugal act as basically resulting from the way God Himself had structured human persons in their bodies.[3] They held that it was a *kind of worship of God* for a person *to accept the basic physical way in which God had formed him or her sexually* and enabled husband and wife to unite sexually. Furthermore, it was *offensive to God* for a person to attempt *to basically take apart the sexual act, so that it would no longer be what God had created.* Indeed such a taking apart would mean that an individual was refusing to be the person which God had made him or her to be.

During the Council, however, some theologians began to show clear signs of holding another, very different version of personalism which we could call *separatist.*[4] This separatist personalism admitted, usually, that our God-given bodily structure and the sexual union which it makes possible were "values." At the same time, separatist thinkers insisted, *the individual could licitly dispense with that structure if he or she conscientiously decided that life would be "more human" without it.* For *true* humanness consisted in actively using one's creative intelligence. On the one hand, this view held, if the natural sexual form of one's body or of the sexual act were creating severe problems in one's life, one could, of course, opt to abstain from sexual actions periodically or even permanently. On the other hand, one could and in some cases perhaps should re-design his or her body or sexual actions. This, according to this second version of personalism, might be preferable to foregoing certain highly valuable, humanizing experiences such as orgasmic sexual union.

The bishops did not, however, deal explicitly with the problem presented by these competing versions of personalism. They were satisfied to make two points: 1) The conjugal act, more than being merely a bodily mechanism for producing a pregnancy, is a *sign;* and 2) The act is a *sign* which *speaks* both of the *mutual love* between husband and wife and of the *procreational nature* of that love.

Married love is an eminently human love because it is an affection between two persons rooted in the will and it embraces the good of the whole person; it can enrich the sentiments of the spirit and *their physical expression* with a unique dignity and ennoble them as the special elements and *signs* of the *friendship* proper to marriage.[5]

Married love is uniquely expressed and perfected *by* the exercise of the *acts proper to marriage*. Hence the *acts* in marriage by which the intimate and chaste union of the spouses takes place are noble and honorable; the truly human performance of *these acts* fosters the self-giving they *signify* and enriches the spouses in joy and gratitude.[6]

One might say, then, that the conjugal act is designed by God not only to generate a *pregnancy*, but also to give a *message*. Indeed, it is the identical message as that found in the wedding vows: "We love each other alone as husband and wife until death, no matter what the cost." The wedding vows can carry this special meaning, of course, only because of their linguistic *structure*. Given the structure which Western civilization builds into its language, one could hardly express wedding vows, for instance, by screaming at one's bride: "I hate you. I can't stand you. And the sooner you die, the better." Nor could one give her a black eye instead of a ring. Certain elements of a civilization's language and symbols are "objective," that is, they are not to be subjected to the whims of those who use them.

In the same way, the Council teaches that *the structure of the conjugal act is not to be subjected to the whims of a couple or an individual.*

Objective criteria must be used, criteria drawn from the nature of the human person and human action, criteria which respect the total *meaning* of mutual self-giving and human procreation in the context of true love: all this is possible only if the virtue of married chastity is seriously practiced.[7]

While the Council did not spell out in further detail what this meant, it did note immediately:

In questions of birth regulation, the sons of the Church, faithful to these principles, are forbidden to use methods disapproved of by the teaching authority of the Church in its interpretation of the divine law.[8]

Attached to this latter statement was a footnote referring to the teachings of previous popes, Pius XI and Pius XII, condemning artificial contraception. Also included in the footnote was a reference to a Commission for the Study of Population, the Family, and Births.[9]

The Papal Commission for the Study of Population, the Family, and Births

The Commission had originally been set up with six members by Pope John XXIII. When Pope Paul VI succeeded Pope John, he expanded it in 1964 to 15 members, and in 1965 to 52 members. Its mandate was to study the need to control family size, particularly from the point of view of morally acceptable means to this end.[10]

The members generally agreed that the Church's teaching on contraception needed to be developed.[11] Most of the members, however, *eventually favored abandoning the teaching of 1900 years* against changing the physical structure of the reproductive system (through contraception sterilization) or of the conjugal act (through contraceptive agents). A minority fought this as *not development, but destruction* of doctrine. The majority denied the charge, though Charles Curran, a leading American opponent of the traditional doctrine, admitted later:

> I in no way mean to impugn the integrity and honesty of those (myself included) who used the theory of historical development to explain how the Catholic Church could change its teaching on artificial contraception.... However, those who argued against the acceptance of artificial contraception in the Roman Catholic Church in the 1960's recognized the more radical nature of the problem.... One must honestly recognize that "the conservatives" saw much more clearly than "the liberals" of the day that a change in the teaching on artificial contraception had to recognize that the previous teaching was wrong.[12]

Moreover, an examination of the proposals which each side submitted shows two extreme opposing positions. On the one hand, the minority defending the official teaching shows great reverence for the conjugal act, but *only* as a bodily mechanism for producing a new life.[13] There is *no hint that the conjugal act is, by its very nature, intended by God to be also a sign of a couple's love* in their mutual giving and accepting of one another in marriage.

On the other hand, the majority opposing the official teaching embraces the separatist version of personalism which we described above: man with his creative intelligence can at times licitly re-design the conjugal act or even his own reproductive system rather than forego orgasmic sexual union.[14] This majority was somewhat restrained in applying the logic of this position. *It was destined to be used within a few years, however, to justify "in certain cases" practically any kind of sexual action, including anal and oral copulation with orgasm, extra-marital relations, masturbation, homosexual actions, and even bestiality.*[15]

The integrist version of personalism does not seem to have attracted the attention of *either faction on the Commission*, and does not appear in the majority's or the minority's final report to the Pope.[16] This is the personalism which, as was noted in Chapter 3, some outstanding theologians developed prior to the Council and which may very well be implicit in the Council documents.

Interestingly enough, *this integrist version of personality was eventually to be accepted as being in harmony with the Biblical faith of the Church* as expressed in Pope Paul VI's letter to the worldwide Church, *Humanae Vitae* (On Human Life) in 1968 and in subsequent Church teaching up to the present time. At the same time, the Church was not to accept the separatist version of personalism, nor was it to find adequate norms which concentrated solely on the procreative power of the conjugal act.

Pope Paul VI's Encyclical

Two years after the Commission's official majority report and its unofficial minority report were submitted to Pope Paul VI, he issued *Humanae Vitae.*[17] His intention to seek an authentically Christian personalist response in this encyclical, and not a physicalist or biologistic one, is evidenced by his words in a General Audience a few days later:

> We willingly followed the personalistic conception that was characteristic of the Council's teaching on conjugal society, thus giving love—which produces that society and nourishes it—the pre-eminent position that rightly belongs to it in a subjective evaluation of marriage.[18]

This orientation of the Pope's teaching is obvious to anyone who seriously studies the encyclical. Sections 7, 8, 9, and 10 are dedicated entirely to an analysis of a couple's basic *decision of love* for one another. Only after this does the Pope proceed to consider the conjugal act. And when he does concentrate on marital acts, it is not only as God-given actions for generating new life, but also and in the first place as God-given *signs* of the *relationship* between husband and wife.

> Nor do these acts cease to be right even if foreseen to be infertile for reasons beyond the control of the married couple, since they do not lose their function of *signifying* and strengthening the deep *relationship* between them.[19] (Emphasis added)

Reference to the *sign*-nature of the conjugal act is frequent throughout the encyclical, in sections 3, 9, and 16, as well as in the central sections 11, 12, and 13. As a matter of fact, the *last* sentence of *section 11* is the oft-quoted condemnation of artificial contraception:

> " . . . Any use of marriage must remain *per se* oriented towards the procreation of human life."

Having reiterated this constant Church teaching, the Pope then proceeds *immediately* in the *first* sentence of *section 12* to give the *reason* for the teaching:

> This doctrine . . . is firmly based on the unbreakable bond established by God between the two *meanings inherent in the act*, namely, unity and procreation.

L. Ciccone's thorough commentary on *Humanae Vitae* notes the importance of the *sequence of thought* at the end of section 11 and the beginning of section 12: *doctrine* followed by *reason for the doctrine. Everything before leads up to this point; everything afterwards depends on it.* Ciccone writes:

> The principle on which the moral evaluation of the conjugal act is founded is no longer whether or not the act is *physically* entire, but whether or not it is a genuine, unaltered, and complete *expression of conjugal love*, which love is by its very nature fruitful, i.e., oriented towards and open to the communication of life.[20] (Emphasis added)

This same principle will be applied later when the Church is forced in the 1970's to confront theologians with dissenting views regarding masturbatory, premarital, and homosexual acts as at times morally licit.

Pope Paul VI, then, broke with the strictly physicalist view of the conjugal act as only an instrument for procreation. It should be noted also that he encouraged couples to seek absolution who, despite their ongoing struggle to respect their conjugal act, sometimes weaken in their resolve and resort to artificial contraception.

> *If, however, sin still exercises its hold over them, they are not to lose heart.* Rather must they, humble and persevering, have recourse to the mercy of God, abundantly bestowed in the Sacrament of Penance. In this way, for sure, they will be able to reach that perfection of married life which the Apostle sets out in these words: "Husbands, love your wives, as Christ loved the Church . . ."[21]

The majority of the Bishops' Conferences throughout the world clearly accepted, presented, explained, and justified the doctrine of *Humanae Vitae.*[22] Some few seemed ambiguous or confusing as they attempted to treat certain individual problems which were not touched on by the encyclical. Several Conferences later cleared up misinterpretations of their words. Two or three at least seem to depart from the Pope's teaching at certain points.

Within days of the release of *Humanae Vitae,* large numbers of theologians, many apparently without having read it, publicly dissented from its teachings. It is difficult, however, to know precisely how many, for the published names of dissenters included many who were in no way professional theologians. Perhaps a majority of theologians in the United States dissented. As possible evidence of this, we might note that *no comprehensive, systematic commentary on* Humanae Vitae *has appeared in English,* whereas there are several in French, German, Italian, and Spanish.

In 1971 and again in 1977 the American Bishops formulated "Ethical and Religious Directives for Catholic Health Facilities" in the face of opposition from leading dissenting theologians, and in 1976 a pastoral letter on the moral life.[23] *Both documents followed the Christian personalistic approach* rooted in the Council's teaching and developed in *Humanae Vitae.* In particular the pastoral on morals reflected the next Vatican document which we will now examine.

" . . . Certain Questions Concerning Sexual Ethics . . . "

The Declaration on Certain Questions Concerning Sexual Ethics was issued by the Sacred Congregation for the Doctrine of the Faith on December 29, 1975.[24] It is a response to a number of theologians who were following out the logic of their separatist version of personalism to justify as licit, at least in certain cases, masturbatory, homosexual, and premarital sexual actions. While *warning Catholics against hasty judgments as to the guilt* of persons who are morally immature, confused, or weak, the Declaration *repudiates all such actions as ever being correct objects of truly human or Christian choice, no matter what the circumstances or the motives.* The basic personalist reason again is that such actions either *in their physical structure* or *in their lack of conjugal commitment* cannot express a true conjugal love.

"Any Sterilization Whatsoever . . . "

In 1975, the same Congregation corroborated the American Bishops' ethical directives forbidding *direct*, that is, *contraceptive* sterilization. Once again the criterion is *personalistic.* For the Congregation does not exclude any and all *physically* direct sterilization, e.g., to protect likely rape victims from impregnation. Rather it condemns all sterilization which seeks to render sterile future sexual actions which a person *intends* to pursue. A person may not licitly *intend* sexual actions, while at the same time only *pretending* that these actions will express a full giving of self in conjugal love.

> Sterilization injures [the] ethical good [of the person] when by deliberate choice it *deprives* of an essential component a sexual act which is *foreseen* and *freely chosen.*[25]

Synod VI and *Familiaris Consortio*

In October 1980, 80 bishops selected by the various national conferences of bishops scattered throughout the world met in Rome for the sixth in a series of Synods of Bishops, with which the Pope consults every three years. This Sixth Synod of Bishops was to concentrate on the family, including its need at times for limiting conceptions.

In December 1981, Pope John Paul II summed up the work of the Synod in a document called *Familiaris Consortio* (On the Family). As is obvious from the following passages *the Holy Father rejects the separatist version of personalism, which would submit the body to any redesigning which man in his "creative intelligence" might deem "more humanizing." The Pope also rejects any merely physicalist or biologistic view of our sexuality.* Instead he

59

blesses a kind of Christian personalism which, in harmony with the Church's biblical faith, sees both man's " *creative intelligence*" and *his physical and sexual structure* as a *gift* which God has carefully created.

Consequently, *sexuality*, by means of which man and woman give themselves to one another through the acts which are proper and exclusive to spouses, is *by no means something purely biological*, but concerns the *innermost being* of the *human person* as such. It is realized in a truly human way only if it is an *integral* part of the love by which a man and a woman commit themselves totally to one another until death.[26] (Emphasis added)

Moreover, the conjugal act enables a man and woman to give themselves to each other precisely because it is *bodily communication* of a *deeply personal message*.

Note how the issue of contraception is treated primarily in terms of *saying* something *true* versus something *false*:

By recourse to contraception, couples separate these two *meanings* which God their Creator has *written* both into their very being as male and female, and into the very forces and energies of their sexual communion. They thus sit in judgement on the plan of God, and twist and degrade human sexuality—and with it themselves and their married partner by undermining its capacity to express total self-giving. Thus they oppose the *natural language* [of the body] which *expresses* total mutual self-giving. They oppose this *language* with another *language* which, through contraception, in objective reality *contradicts* [what they should want to say to one another]. For the structure of the contraceptive *act says* that they do not want to give themselves totally to one another. This leads not only to a positive refusal to be open to life, but also to a *falsification* of the *truth* which is the heart of the love of a husband and wife. For this love calls for giving one's whole person.

In contrast to this, by recourse to periods of infertility, a couple respects the inseparable connection between the unitive and procreative *meanings* of human sexuality. They thus act as stewards of God's plan and use their sexuality according to its original force and energy for total self-giving, without *pretence* or alteration.[27] (Emphasis added)

60

Sex, A Highly *Personal* Thing

A theologian who is truly Catholic always works within the unity of the Church as the living visible body of the Lord Jesus. This means that, of necessity, he ultimately submits his work, not only to the discernment of his academic peers, but also to that of the whole body of the Church. This, in turn, means that he submits his work to the judgement of the Bishops who, united through the ministry of Peter and his successors, are servants of that body's unity in truth.

This chapter has shown how these Bishops, in the 20th century, have sifted through the work of theologians, and discerned there what is of authentic service to Christian faith and life. They have affirmed that sex is for persons only, *persons* who *like* being the *persons* whom God has formed, soul and body, by His hand and in His image.

Discussion Questions

1. Who was Pope John XXIII? What is generally people's attitude towards him as he is remembered? Did he give any specific teaching regarding sexual morality?
2. In what sense is sexual union designed by God to be a "personalist act?"
3. What two incompatible versions of personalism emerged during the period of the Second Vatican Council?
4. Did the Council teach that one could be a good Catholic and nonetheless reject the Church's teaching on contraception?
5. Did the rejection of the Church's traditional teaching on contraception turn out to be a radical move?
6. Why do we call the Church's personalistic approach to sexuality "integrist?"

Notes

1. *The Pope Speaks*, 1962, Vol. 7, p. 331.
2. *The Pope Speaks*, 1963, Vol. 9, p. 21.
3. See John Noonan, *Contraception: A History of its Treatment by the Catholic Theologians and Canonists*, (Cambridge, Harvard, 1965) pp. 491–504. Cf. William May for the terminology, "integrist" and "separatist," in *Dimensions of Human Sexuality*, ed. Dennis Doherty (Garden City, Doubleday, 1979) pp. 95–124.
4. See the "Argument for Reform" in Peter Harris *et. al.*, *On Human Life, An Examination of Humanae Vitae*, (London, Burns and Oats, 1968), pp. 206–207.
5. No. 49 in Vatican Council II, *The Conciliar and Post-Conciliar Documents*, ed. Austin Flannery, O.P., (Northport, Costello, 1975), p. 952.
6. *Ibid.*

7. *Ibid.*, no. 51, p. 955, emphasis added.

8. *Ibid.*

9. *Ibid.*

10. Noonan, *op. cit.*, p. 531, footnote 113.

11. "The Minority Working Paper," in Harris *el. al., op. cit.*, pp. 175–202, especially pp. 181, 198, and 201.

12. "Ten Years Later," in *Commonweal*, July 7, 1978, p. 426.

13. "The Minority Working Paper," *op. cit., passim*, but esp. pp. 177–180, and 197–198.

14. "Argument for Reform," *op. cit.*, pp. 206–207.

15. Michael Valente, *Sex: The Radical View of a Catholic Theologian* (New York, Bruce, 1970), pp. 115–155, especially pp. 130–140. Valente's book is cited with approval at least as to the essential elements or "values" of sexual activities in the Catholic Theological Society of America's controversial study, Anthony Kosnick *et. al. Human Sexuality: New Directions in American Catholic Thought*, (New York, Paulist, 1977), pp. 92, 261–262, 270.

16. In Harris, *op. cit.*, pp. 216–244.

17. *Humanae Vitae* in *The Pope Speaks*, Vol. 13, pp. 329–346.

18. *Ibid.* p. 207.

19. *Humanae Vitae*, no. 11.

20. L. Ciccone "L'Encylica Humanae Vitae: Analisi E Commento," in *Divus Thomas*, Piancenza, 1969, p. 271.

21. *Humanae Vitae, op. cit.*, no. 25.

22. Marcellino Zalba, "The Magisterium of the Pope and the Episcopal Conferences," in *Natural Family Planning* (Milwaukee, De Rance, 1980), pp. 215–223.

23. *Ethical and Religious Directives for Catholic Health Facilities* (Washington, United States Catholic Conference, 1971 and 1977); and *To Live in Christ Jesus*, (same publisher, 1976).

24. *The Declaration on Certain Questions in Concerning Sexual Ethics*, (Washington, United States Catholic Conference, 1976).

25. *Commentary on Reply of the Sacred Congregation for the Doctrine of the Faith on Sterilization in Catholic Hospitals* (Washington, United States Catholic Conference, 1978), nos. 1 and 3.

26. In *Origins*, Vol. 11, nos. 28 and 29, December 24, 1981, n. 11.

27. *Ibid.*, n. 32., slightly edited.

Preview of
Chapter Six

● The secular sexual ethics portrayed in the media as modern and scientific derives from a view of human sexuality as developed in a purposeless process of biological evolution.

● Christian sexual ethics embraces both the animal and the rational aspects of the human person and sexuality.

● The procreative and unitive values of human sexuality are ethically inseparable by human choice because their combination comes not from mere evolution but from God's wise provision for human good.

● The act of conjugal intercourse is the natural sacrament and effective sign of the deeper spiritual love of husband and wife.

● Specific sexual norms reject sexual pleasure separated from love, sexual love separated from the family, and procreation separated from sexual love.

● A controversial approach to moral norms called ethical proportionalism offers the possibility of finding exceptions in applying all sexual norms; it is not recommended.

CHAPTER 6

Sexual Norms in Catholic Teaching

The Catholic vision of human sexuality presented from a historical perspective in Chapters 1 through 3 and from the perspective of recent Church teachings in the last chapter may seem as outdated as the horse and buggy and outdoor bathroom facilities to some people. Why? The challenges described in Chapter 4 offer a partial explanation.

Secular humanism and its version of secular ethics accompany these challenges throughout the world, especially in nations enjoying the advancing technology and scientific research of Western civilization. Many proponents of secular sexual ethics have long since abandoned the pivotal norm of Catholic sexual morality, that human genital activity cannot be morally good unless it expresses the interpersonal relationship of marriage. These influential thinkers and opinion-makers of the Western world *have not considered the stable family a major objective of society, as it is in a social order shaped by a Christian vision.*

A 1983 study on leadership attitudes by the American Enterprise Institute for Public Policy Research interviewed 104 top executives and TV writers in the U.S. entertainment world. It found that two-thirds earn more than $200,000 annually. The same proportion admitted that they attempt to move their audience "toward their own vision of the good society." In that vision only 49% of them see adultery as wrong, 20% rate homosexual actions wrong, and 3% oppose abortion.[1]

Active Christians are often a powerless minority throughout the modern world. Their view of sexual ethics is made to appear outmoded and impractical in the face of the view presented as scientific and modern by powerful opinion-makers who claim to represent the majority of intelligent and enlightened persons.

Unfortunately, many viewers of television entertainment are unaware that the secular sexual ethics so often portrayed there differs radically from Christian doctrine. They presume that somehow Christianity *has already* or *soon will* accommodate itself to this sexual ethics which is pictured as *truly modern and correct.*

Only two sexual norms seem morally binding in this secular sexual ethics:

1) Social attitudes or laws are unjust if they hinder human freedom to achieve sexual values in whatever way the individual desires—as long as no other person is harmed.
2) Sexual behavior among consenting adults is entirely a matter to be determined by personal choice.

These two norms of secular sexual ethics derive from the vision of sexuality in which human sexuality developed simply by accident through the purposeless process of biological evolution. The ethics of radical individualism which holds that society exists only to protect one individual from another is a second source of the above two sexual norms.

Yet the same *basic values of human sexuality and human sexual relationships* are experienced by Christians and secular humanists alike. Christian sexual norms are rooted in that experience as interpreted in the light of God's revelation. This chapter will explore the ethical basis of Catholic sexual norms and the current controversy within the field of Catholic sexual ethics about making exceptions to universal moral norms.

Human Persons and Their Sexual Nature

The classical description of a human person as a *rational animal* indicates that each human being enjoys both biological and intellectual existence simultaneously and in a unified manner. The term "animal" refers to bodily existence and the complex physical, chemical, and biological structure of the body. The term "rational" refers to very complex human behavior based on abstract knowledge and manifesting a freedom that transcends the instinctive life of animals.

All human persons belong to a single, interacting human community in which they not only eat, drink, and reproduce (as animals do), but also think scientifically and creatively, debate and make decisions, and make love (as only rational individuals can do). Human persons need and create community for survival and for human fulfillment in communication and love.

Erroneous views of the human person exaggerate either the animal or the rational aspect of human existence. *Biologism* or *physicalism* identifies human nature with the physical structure and biological drives of the human body. This reduces human persons to animals for whom the good life is lived purely according to biological instincts in a completely determined way. The opposite view, which might be called *reconstructionism*, identifies human nature with creative reason, claiming the right to ignore the biological structure of human beings and reconstruct the self uniquely according to personal choice. (This latter view is reflected in the separatist personalism discussed in the previous chapter.)

Christian ethics embraces what is .true in both these extreme positions since the human person combines both aspects of human existence. Christians view this world and themselves as gifts of God. They accept from Him the responsibility of stewardship over human life, health, and sexuality.

Christians also recognize that persons of vastly different cultural and historical backgrounds *enjoy a common human nature, even though at any given moment of history the moral insights and ethical convictions of any group of persons is profoundly conditioned by their history.*

Yet in order to have a history and a culture, human persons must, and actually do, have this common mode of existence as the authentic source of human action and achievement. One aspect of that common human nature is under discussion in this book: The sexuality of human persons.

Human sexuality affects every aspect of human existence. The Vatican *Declaration on Certain Questions Concerning Sexual Ethics* of 1975 suggested that "It is from sex that the human person receives the characteristics which, on the biological, psychological and spiritual levels, make that person a man or a woman, and thereby largely condition his or her progress toward maturity and insertion into society."[2]

Fathers Ashley and O'Rourke in their volume, *Health Care Ethics*, list these four chief categories of the values of human sexuality.[3]

1) Sex is a *search for sensual pleasure* and satisfaction, releasing physical and psychic tensions.
2) Sex is a *search for the completion of the human person* through and in intimate *personal union* of love expressed by bodily union.
3) Sex is a *social necessity for the procreation and education of children* in the family to expand the human community.
4) Sex is a *religious mystery*, somehow revealing the cosmic order.

These basic values are generally recognized in ethical theories about sexuality because they are matters of common human experience. Fathers Ashley and O'Rourke point out, though, two important insights added by the Christian tradition.

First, these values of sexuality are ethically *inseparable* by human choice, because their combination is not the result of mere evolution, but of God's wise provision for human good. Second, the religious value of sex is that it provides an *experience of love* which teaches people the meaning of other kinds of love, especially the love between God and the human community.[4]

The second insight suggests that sexual love and its cultivation in the marital relationship should not be seen as an absolute good but a relative good. It means that human persons are fulfilled through lives of love, but conjugal love is not an indispensable form of human love.

In the Judeo-Christian tradition and particularly in Catholic teaching, the moral norms applicable to human sexuality have especially come from the first insight just mentioned, the inseparable connections of the basic values of human sexuality.

Sexuality as Procreative and Unitive

As a result, the procreative purpose of sexual intercourse has been emphasized throughout the long history of Church teaching. Without procreation, the human race would obviously perish in a few years! The biological sciences have shown advantages of sexual reproduction over asexual reproduction as a means of preserving living species and promoting their evolution to better adapted forms of life.

But human sexual procreation differs from animal reproduction. The man and woman who procreate are persons, not animals, and God creates in and through their procreative act. When a child is conceived, the child is also a member of the human family, not merely an animal. *Catholic teaching holds that God acts in a creative way through the procreative act of parents so that the newly conceived person enjoys a relationship to Him and an eternal destiny as all persons do.*

The behavioral sciences reveal that the basic pattern in which human persons have exercised their procreative gift is that of monogamous marriage. This makes sense in view of two facts of human biology: 1) the time of human gestation and child care is remarkably long, no doubt, to aid development of the complex human brain and to teach basic behavioral patterns to the child; 2) sexual intercourse is not confined to a mating season but ties man and woman in a lasting bond assuring the mother that the man will share her burden of child care as father.

The need for continuous companionship of the father with his wife and children has necessitated the social institution of the family. The chief cultural alternative to monogamy has been polygyny, one father with many wives, which diminishes the equality of women with men and is impractical for most men.

In fact, the human desire for completion through love expressed in bodily union indicates *another value and meaning which God has given to human sexuality. The love of man and woman as a personal bond of life does not arise merely from biological attraction to sensual pleasure.* It arises culturally and historically out of the institution of the family. The bonding of man to woman seems to have its evolutionary explanation in the needs of large-brained human children and their rearing. One cannot scientifically explain this bonding as separate from, or more human than, the procreative function of human sexuality.

The love bonding of man and woman extends itself to their children as the overflowing of that love. Human procreation fulfills not just a blind instinct or a compulsive drive for pleasure, but a free act of commitment to love one another in a bodily union open to the future through procreation.

Through the family, God achieves His ultimate purpose of creating a vast family of persons to enter eternal community with the Trinity in mutual knowledge and love. The true personal love between husband and wife is part of the ultimate goal of the universe and not merely a means of continuing the human species.

The act of conjugal intercourse is the natural sacrament and effective sign of the deeper spiritual love of husband and wife. God Himself designed this sign of total mutual self-giving. Through experiencing the rich satisfactions of conjugal love which are physical, psychological, and interpersonal, spouses learn to transcend their egoism and grow in Christian love.

Couples blessed with children learn from educating their children to be more human themselves. Conjugal sexuality is not completed in sexual orgasm but in begetting and raising a family. Those who grow old without children find it hard to keep their love alive and attain full maturity. If couples are unable to have children, this privation can, fortunately, be spiritually overcome if it is accepted as part of the mystery of the Cross as taught by Jesus.

Previous chapters of this book have surveyed the ways in which Catholic theology and Church teaching have presented sexual morality. The inseparability of the procreative and unitive meanings of sexual intercourse has led to specific moral norms that distinguish sexual activity which is morally good from that which is not.

Specific Sexual Norms

These sexual norms in the Judeo-Christian tradition focus on, 1) *sexual pleasure separated from love*, 2) *sexual love separated from the family*, and 3) *procreation separated from sexual love*. In every case these norms proscribe sexual activity which distorts its own inherent meaning and purpose and hence in a very real sense deforms the human person. These traditional norms are reviewed here very briefly.

The first set of norms judges morally wrong *all sexual actions whose purpose is not the expression of love but the seeking of sexual pleasure or the release of sexual tension apart from the expression of love*. This includes both normal acts of heterosexual intercourse of unmarried persons and homosexual acts when either are performed primarily for sexual excitement. It also includes masturbation, sexual activity with animals, and various forms of abnormal sexual behavior including indulgence in pornography and deliberate sexual fantasy for the sake of genital excitement. Some sociological studies have suggested that such acts do no physical or psychological harm, but they do harm the integrity of the persons involved. It might also be noted that if pornography does no harm neither do the fine arts do any good. Hence these acts can be described as depersonalizing.

Moreover, the pursuit of pleasure for its own sake becomes obsessive or addictive and injures human freedom. Alcohol and drug addiction dramatically manifest this but sex is no less obsessive. The pursuit of pleasure exclusively for its own sake leads to more and more aberrant behavior and then to boredom, depression, and despair. One can show that human pleasure becomes humanly satisfying only when it accompanies the achievement of some more permanent good like health, friendship, or love.

The second set of norms judges morally wrong *all sexual actions which separate sexual love from the family.* This means that despite loving intentions, the following sexual acts are morally wrong: acts of sexual intercourse between unmarried persons, adulterous actions, genital activity expressing a homosexual relationship, and contraceptive acts which eliminate the procreative significance of marital intercourse.

Many of the actions mentioned here spring from human efforts to approach the ideal of sexual love in the face of various conflicts and tensions. Church teaching has always recognized a variety of circumstances in which a person is not totally responsible for such acts or may even act in subjective good faith. But it has insisted that such actions are gravely opposed to the meaning and purpose of human genital activity and contrary to the integrity of human persons as persons.

The third set of norms judges morally wrong *those forms of artificial reproduction of human persons which actually separate procreation from sexual love.* Artificial insemination of a wife with sperm from a donor clearly creates this separation, but even artificial insemination with a husband's sperm separates procreation from sexual love.

Father Benedict Ashley, O.P., a Catholic theologian writing on medical ethics, points out that such technologies, which include the more recently developed procedure of "test-tube" fertilization, violate the child's right to have "parents in the strict sense."[5] The subjective attitude of the parents who deeply long for a child cannot substitute for the objective relation of the child to its parents. To loosen the conception of the child from its direct relation to the sacramental act of love which is normal conjugal intercourse diminishes the child's security.

Part two of this book will discuss in greater depth the issues of contraception, homosexual activity, and technological reproduction. However, in the contemporary discussion of all these practices a central and essential issue of ethical analysis emerges. Must the traditional Catholic teaching on the inherent evil of the acts violating these specific sexual norms be maintained? Are these moral norms to apply without exception, or can a combination of extenuating circumstances and compensating values create exceptions in which such behavior should not be considered morally evil?

Proportionalism and Sexual Norms

The trend of much ethical reflection in the twentieth century has been to emphasize the dynamic and developing aspects of human morality. Existentialism is a trend in modern philosophy which has emphasized the key role of free and personal decision in establishing the way a person's behavior reflects his or her personality and vice versa.

This led to considerable doubt about the exceptionless character of the sexual moral norms just reviewed. The birth control issue of the twentieth century already described in this book focused particular attention on the norm which judges contraception in conjugal intercourse an immoral act.

The classical theory taught in Catholic sexual ethics holds that the contracepted act of conjugal intercourse has become evil because the intervention eliminated the procreative meaning of the act.

While the ways of supporting this judgment have varied with different ethicists and their interpretations of the precise evil of contraception, all agreed that the act had become destructive of the good of the person and evil in itself. Hence spouses using contraception were judged to perform moral evil, regardless of good intentions and marital pressures, and even if the persons had reduced culpability or acted in good faith.

In the 60's there gradually evolved a moral theory called *proportionalism.* It holds that the moral evil in such acts should not be designated moral evil until the circumstances and intention of the person acting are taken into account. These acts would still clearly oppose the full meaning of conjugal intercourse, so a term was necessary to recognize this evil aspect of the acts. The two terms which were coined are "premoral evil" or "ontic evil." The latter term, coming from the Greek word for "being," designates the reality of the evil without at the same time invoking the notion of moral evil.

All agree that the term *moral evil* applies to those evils which hinder the true goal of human moral life. *The essential thesis of proportionalism proposes that, in certain cases, the evil of conjugal contraception should not be designated as moral evil.* Instead, extenuating circumstances and other benefits of the contracepted act may outweigh the evil, allowing it to be simply designated premoral or ontic evil.

An author who consistently applies this methodology to sexual activity is the Sulpician, Father Philip S. Keane. His summary statement on contraception says this:

> If a couple face serious medical, psychological, or economic problems, their need for the human values involved in sexual communion would seem to give moral justification to their use of birth control devices. Such a decision by a couple will be undertaken with some regret (due to the ontically evil elements in birth control), but with a good conscience and with the conviction that, all things being considered, their action is objectively moral.[6]

71

Father Keane uses the same methodology to justify sexual intercourse in some instances where an unmarried couple are deeply committed to each other and fully intend to marry, as well as instances of homosexual activity and masturbation.[7] In all cases, he maintains that exceptions depend on a prudent judgment of all circumstances and that the method does not give a license for overthrowing traditional sexual morality.

In fact, some who use this method of proportionalism are so sensitive to the social importance of sexual norms that in instances like the morality of sexual intercourse without a marital covenant they support the traditional prohibition as "virtually exceptionless." But they generally are very tolerant of marital contraception which they justify for the unitive stability and happiness of the spouses.

Subsequent chapters of this book will explore further the applications of this method of ethical proportionalism. But the editors of this book do not themselves adopt or recommend this method. They object to it as contrary to an authentic understanding of the moral significance of human sexual behavior as well as certain other behavior where human actions directly violate human rights or the life and dignity of persons. (Abortion is a prime example of this.) They also believe that it undermines the Church's moral doctrine and her understanding of the human person and key areas of moral activity.

Objections to Proportionalism

Several competent Catholic ethicists have recently published scholarly essays objecting to ethical proportionalism in the key areas of human behavior just described.[8] Perhaps the two most basic arguments of these authors are as follows. First, they insist on the incorrectness of using the terms "ontic" or "premoral" to describe the evil in the actions violating the sexual norms discussed here. Secondly, they argue that once this qualification has been introduced, no rational method remains for measuring the proportion of values and non-values to decide whether the act should be judged morally evil.

Father Servais Pinckaers, O.P., a professor at the University of Fribourg, Switzerland, recently published a profound study which tends to support the first point raised here.[9] He points out the error of supposing that actions like those which undermine the meaning and purpose of human sexuality might in some cases involve only ontic or premoral, and not moral evil.

Father Pinckaers insists that, by rejecting the notion of intrinsic morality, proportionalism reduces morality to a merely technical question of the most effective way of attaining ends extrinsic to the human person.

It ignores the fact that every free human act first of all affects the integrity of the actor, making him or her more or less truly human. *Thus the person who performs a sexual act contradictory to the authentic meaning of human sexuality in that very act, apart from the attainment of any further values, distorts his or her own personality.* **He shows that this approach to morality is the outcome of the very legalism it attempts to mitigate.**

Fathers Ashley and O'Rourke have discussed the second objection to proportionalism, the problem of measuring and weighing the so-called ontic aspects of human actions independently of their moral significance.[10] They point out that to consider the ontic aspects of a human act apart from their relation to the true end of human life deprives them of any value or disvalue which is morally relevant. But if that were the case, there would be no point of reference for weighing or comparing the value and disvalue.

This very serious controversy about the exceptionless character of basic sexual norms challenges ethicists in the Catholic tradition to further dialogue and clarification. The implications of this controversy for the moral analysis of contraception, homosexuality, and technological reproduction will surface in Chapters 10, 15, and 17.

Discussion Questions

1. What are the two basic norms of a secular sexual ethics and where do they come from?
2. What are the four chief categories of sexual values in common human experience?
3. What religious significance is found in the term procreation?
4. Why does an evolutionary explanation of the love bonding of man and woman relate it to the needs of large-brained human children?
5. What are the three sets of specific sexual norms reviewed in this chapter?
6. What is the difference between ethical proportionalism and the tradition of basic exceptionless moral norms?
7. How might you relate the notion of exceptionless moral norms to the nature of the human person and his or her actions?

Notes

1. *Crux of the News*. March 7, 1983 (Albany, N.Y., Gabriel Publishing Company).
2. *Declaration on Certain Questions Concerning Sexual Ethics*. Vatican Congregation for the Doctrine of the Faith, Dec. 29, 1975, #1.
3. Ashley, Benedict M., and O'Rourke, Kevin D., *Health Care Ethics: A Theological Analysis*, (St. Louis, MO., The Catholic Health Assoc., 2nd Edit., 1982) pp. 205–06.

4. *Ibid.* p. 206.

5. Ashley, Benedict M., "A Child's Right to His Own Parents: A Look at Two Value Systems," *Hospital Progress.* 61 (Aug., 1980) pp. 47–49.

6. Keane, Philip S., *Sexual Morality. A Catholic Perspective.* (New York, N.Y., Paulist Press, 1977) p. 125 The book originally was certified by a bishop with his imprimatur as being reasonably defensible by Catholic standards; but this imprimatur was revoked in 1985. For a sympathetic description of ethical proportionalism, see McKeever, Rev. Paul E., "Proportionalism as a Methodology in Catholic Moral Theology", in *Human Sexuality and Personhood* (St. Louis, MO, Pope John Center, 1981), pp. 211–22. For a more thorough and technical presentation, see: McCormick, Richard A. and Ramsey, Paul, eds. *Doing Evil to Achieve Good: Moral Choice in Conflict Situations.* (Chicago, Loyola University Press, 1978). Rev. Richard A. McCormick supports this methodology in his annual review article on moral theology in *Theological Studies.* Cf., for example, "Notes on Moral Theology: 1981", *Theological Studies,* 43:1, Mar., 1982, pp. 69–91.

7. *Ibid.* pp. 107, 87, 67.

8. Connery, John R., "Catholic Ethics: Has the Norm for Rule-Making Changed?," *Theological Studies.* 42, June, 1981, pp. 232–250; May, William E., "Roman Catholic Ethics and Beneficence," in *Beneficence and Health Care.* ed. by Earl E. Shelp, (Holland: Reidel Publ, Kluwer Boston, 1982), pp. 127–52; Grisez, Germain G., "Christian Moral Theology and Consequentialism", in *Principles of Catholic Moral Life.* ed. by William E. May, (Chicago: Franciscan Herald Press, 1980), pp. 293–328; Lee Patrick, "Permanence of the Ten Commandments: St. Thomas and his Modern Commentators," *Theological Studies.* 42:3, 1981, pp. 422–43.

9. Pinckaers, Servais, "La Question des Actes Intrinsequement Mauvais et le 'Proportionalism'", *Revue Thomiste.* 82, Ap-June, 1982, pp. 181–212. Ed note: Fr. Pinckaers makes a distinction between the moral finality and a finality of a technical type which organizes means to an end on the basis of usefulness. This distinction seems to be rooted in the classic distinction of Aristotle between prudence as governing upright activity regarding human goods, and "art" (GR. *techné*) as governing every type of making or production. (Cf. Aristotle, *Nichomachean Ethics.* Bk. vi, chap. 4–5.)

10. Ashley and O'Rourke, *op. cit..* pp. 169–170.

Preview of
Chapter Seven

• The Church needs to be able to depend on Christian families for much of the evangelization She needs to do in present-day society.

• Human procreation surpasses mere animal reproduction in that the parents provide the occasion for a creative act of God.

• Divine Providence brings two people together to form a home; this is the "beginning" of their vocation to marriage and the family.

• Children are a gift from God to the spouses, to the Church, and to society.

• Seeing Christian marriage as a call from God to a man and a woman to realize something great underscores their need for help:

• from each other: to overcome their defects, to grow in the virtues, and to raise their children "in wisdom and age and grace";

• from the Church: for the grace of the sacraments, the support and stimulus of Her authentic teachings, and for counsel in making decisions;

• from society: to never oppose, but rather support the unity of the family, to supplement the efforts of the parents to form and educate their children, and to provide financial and other aids meant to assist parents to overcome undue obstacles to achieving their formative task;

- from God: to maintain ever young in fidelity their love for one another and their vision of the lofty goal of Christian sanctity.

CHAPTER 7

The Christian Vocation of Marriage

Divorce, concubinage, cultic prostitution, homosexuality and bisexuality, contraception, abortion, infanticide—all these practices figured prominently among the sins denounced by St. Paul (cf. Rom 1, 18–32; 1 Cor 6, 9–10 inter alia). He also dealt with the rationalizations and justifications of such practices supplied by the cultural and intellectual leaders of the day. St. Paul presents these practices as a "chastisement" by God for the pagan failure to be faithful to the insights of their more astute thinkers, although even the great pagan philosophers condescended to one or another of such evils. In any case, the new members of the young Christian religion saw it as part of their very vocation "in Christ" to restore human dignity to the social customs of the day.

Human history has once again brought us to a social situation where all of the above evils are once again found prospering. Many persons today no longer view marriage in a Christian way, but have reverted to a vision more in accord with the pagan views of other times and places. Christians are once again living amidst a plurality of viewpoints regarding marriage, man's nature, the existence of God and the importance of morality. They experience confusion over which—if any—of these views are compatible with the fundamental Christian outlook on life, particularly when their sense of Christian vocation is inadequate or non-existent.

There is today no lack of intellectual justification for the acceptance of customs and practices long considered intrinsically evil by Christians. Particularly in this century, with the "maturing" of the social sciences (especially economics, psychology and sociology), marriage as an ideal and an institution has been under sustained assault. In the last decade or so, some social scientists seem to be reacting against the unscientific character of many of the critiques and/or theories upon which many anti-marriage and anti-family attacks have relied,[1] but at present it is impossible to see where this development will lead.

In 1972 the Cardinal Archbishop of Krakow, Karol Wojtyla, wrote a book dedicated to "the implementation of Vatican II."[2] His premise in the book is that the "pastoral" nature of the recent Council's magisterium seeks a different response from the faithful than past "dogmatic" Councils. Instead of seeking "religious assent of mind," he perceives it to be the desire of the Second Vatican Council to elicit an enrichment of faith in truths proclaimed, recalled, and further clarified "for the primary purpose of giving Christians a life-style, a way of thinking and acting." This enrichment of human existence through an enrichment of Christian faith would show itself in a deeper and more perceptive *consciousness* of the truths of Revelation, as well as through more appropriate *attitudes* among the faithful toward those same truths, and their practical implications for human action.[3]

In this Chapter we have adopted a similar scheme. First, we intend to present the ideal of marriage and the family, proposed by the Church as true "vocational" realities in the Church and in society. It will then be shown that this consciousness illustrates the need for formation or training in the virtues and attitudes necessary for spouses to have any chance of attaining such an ideal. It also implies that this training is never entirely complete, since it includes the commitment to be a disciple of Christ; to seek sanctity, a lifetime work.

I. Christian Consciousness of Marriage and the Family

Marriage is a Human and Christian Vocation

All living things reproduce themselves. One of the ways in which the generation of a species occurs is through sexual reproduction. Biologists tell us that there is an advantage to sexual forms of reproduction over asexual ones. Sexual reproduction offers greater rapidity with which new genetic combinations are formed among individuals of the species in question:

> To diversify is to adapt; sexually reproducing populations are more likely than asexual ones to create new genetic combinations better adjusted to changed conditions in the environment. Asexual forms are permanently committed to their particular combinations and are more likely to become extinct when the environment fluctuates.[4]

That the human race also reproduces itself, and through sexual intercourse, is a fact; to ignore this fact would be both theological and scientific dishonesty. The "advantages" of which the biologists speak in this context, however, are evolutionary advantages of primary benefit to the *species*, albeit through the "fitness" of individuals to bear up under environmental stress. In this view, reproduction is not a moral act, and it is certainly not a "vocation;" it is merely a fact of biological existence.

If man were defined only as an animal which reproduces sexually, then marriage and the family could be dismissed simply as highly adaptive modes of behavior designed to ensure the survival of the species. Clearly man is more than this. Philosophy, theology, literature, and many other fields of learning point to that other, greater, more fascinating part of the human being: the soul.

The human soul, since it is immaterial, cannot be produced from any pre-existent material. It must be created every time a new human person comes into existence. Creation *ex nihilo* ("from nothingness") is an act which only God can perform, since it requires an infinite active power which no creature can possess.[5] From a Christian viewpoint, marriage is the state in which it is appropriate for a man and a woman to cooperate with God in the creation of a human being. In a very real sense, each child resulting from human procreation is *a gift from God*, entrusted to both the husband and the wife *together*, for its further human and spiritual development. It has been said that

> being a father or a mother is not simply a matter of bringing children into the world. The capacity for generation, which is a share in the creative power of God, is meant to have a continuation. Parents are called to cooperate with the Holy Spirit in the development of their children into men and women

who will be authentic Christians. The parents are the first persons responsible for the education of their children, in human as well as in spiritual matters. They should be conscious of the extent of their responsibility.[6]

This Christian point of view brings out clearly the whole vocational context within which married life and the family must be seen. These principles apply equally to non-Christian couples who must raise their children according to the truth as perceived by them in conscience.

The Catholic Church sees human beings according to a new, revealed mode: They are members of the "supernatural" race of the children of God in the New Man, Jesus Christ.[7] The object of the Church's care and concern is

> man in his unique unrepeatable human reality, which keeps intact the image and likeness of God Himself. The Council points out this very fact when, speaking of that likeness, it recalls that "man is the only creature on earth that God willed for itself" (*Gaudium et spes*, #24). Man as "willed" by God, as "chosen" by Him for eternity and called, destined for grace and glory—this is "each" man, "the most concrete" man, "the most real"; this is man in all the fullness of the mystery in which he has become a sharer in Jesus Christ, the mystery in which each one of the four thousand million human beings living on our planet has become a sharer from the moment he is conceived beneath the heart of his mother.[8]

Christ indicates His will for each and every one of us both directly and indirectly through others (persons, things and events). This is Divine Providence manifesting itself to each individual as a "calling" or "vocation."

Christian marriage is a true vocation in the Church. Christian couples, and those who counsel them, should see Christian marriage integrated within the universal call to sanctity of the entire People of God:

> For a Christian marriage is not just a social institution, much less a mere remedy for human weakness. It is a real supernatural calling. A great sacrament, in Christ and in the Church, says St. Paul (Eph 5, 32). . . . Husband and wife are called to sanctify their married life and to sanctify themselves in it. It would be a serious mistake if they were to exclude family life from their spiritual development. The marriage union, the care and education of children, the effort to pro-

vide for the needs of the family as well as for its security and development, the relationships with other persons who make up the community, all these are among the ordinary human situations that Christian couples are called upon to sanctify.[9]

Christian couples should never forget that through the sacrament of Matrimony they are possessed of a special *charism*, the grace of the sacrament, which is a promise of the Lord to assist them in the trials and difficulties arising from their state. This grace, then, is a special help that they may live out their vocations in fidelity to the Lord.

The Christian family is of great significance for the life and health of the whole Body of Christ. The striving of the family members after sanctity through the exercise of charity and the other virtues contributes to the spiritual development of the Church through the Communion of Saints. Children are a gift from God not only to the couple who begot them but also to the Church. Vatican II was only repeating an idea traditional in the Church since St. Augustine when it observed:

> From the marriage of Christians there comes the family in which new citizens of human society are born and, by the grace of the Holy Spirit in Baptism, those are made children of God so that the People of God may be perpetuated throughout the centuries.[10]

Through the often heroic example of their lives, and through their training of the children in Christian doctrine and living, they prepare them to eventually assume mature and responsible roles in society and in the Church.

The Sacrament of Marriage

The Church's traditional consciousness with regard to marriage is expressed by the oft-quoted statement that "matrimony among baptized persons is a sacrament." This expression indicates that the Church holds not only that true matrimony can and does exist for non-Christians but also that there is some special significance to Christian marriage. Here, we address both of these perceptions.

a) Marriage is a Natural Reality

The generation and propagation of the human race would appear to be subject to much the same natural necessity which governs other biological beings. This thought is well expressed by the biblical writer who relates the divine mandate: "Be fertile and multiply; fill the earth. . . ." (Gn 1, 28) However, there is also something "special" about human reproduction, or more exactly, human "procreation;" this is attested to not only by the endless variety of elaborate ceremonies "celebrating" marriage, but also by Sacred Writ: "The man had relations with his wife Eve, and she conceived and bore Cain, saying, 'I have produced a man *with the help of the Lord.*'" (Gn 4, 1; cf. 4, 25)

We have stated in a previous section that the generation of a human child is really the cooperation by the parents with an act of God, the creative act. The child is truly a gift; a gift of God, not to one or the other, but to both parents as a unit. The child's upbringing, if it is truly to become a mature, responsible and virtuous human being, must be carried out by its parents in a fittingly human manner. This is so because a true "education" is a "leading-out" of all the human qualities which a human child possesses potentially. At the very least, then, it can be said that to the extent that the child is incapable of accomplishing this for itself there is a "natural" (of *human* nature) need for marriage and the family.

b) The Christian Marriage is an Ecclesial Reality

The sacraments of the Church are outward signs instituted by Christ to give grace. They signify or symbolize some reality, and actually effect what they signify. For example, in Baptism a person is "washed" with water to signify the cleansing of the soul which the sacrament is actually bringing about.

Matrimony was formally defined as a sacrament at the Council of Trent (1545–1563). That Council taught that

> since matrimony under the law of the gospel is, because of the grace given through Christ, superior to the marriage unions of earlier times, our holy Fathers, the councils, and the tradition of the universal Church have always rightly taught that matrimony should be included among the sacraments of the New Law.[11]

Christ, in elevating human marriage to sacramental status, did so in view of the unity which God had established should exist between man and wife *from the beginning,* that is, from before sin's entrance into the world.

Have you not read that at the beginning the creator made them male and female and declared, "For this reason a man shall leave his father and mother and cling to his wife, and the two shall become as one"? Thus they are no longer two but one flesh. Therefore, let no man separate what God has united. (Mt 19, 4–6)

The coming together of *this* man and *this* woman to offer and accept one another in an attitude of complete self-giving is not a mere human caprice, but rather a union planned and willed by God, a "great mystery." Sacramentality, strictly speaking, does not change the reality of human marriage itself in any way, but rather elevates its symbolic content by making it explicitly Christ-centered, and by making it productive of Grace.

What, then, is the sign of the sacrament of matrimony? The following words from *Familiaris consortio* are clear regarding the sign-content of Christian marriage:

The communion between God and His people finds its definitive fulfillment in Jesus Christ, the Bridegroom who loves and gives Himself as the Savior of humanity, uniting it to Himself as His body. He reveals the original truth of marriage, the truth of the "beginning" (cf. Gn 2, 24; Mt 19, 5), and, freeing man from his hardness of heart, He makes man capable of realizing this truth in its entirety. This revelation reaches its definitive fullness in the gift of love which the Word of God makes to humanity in assuming a human nature, and in the sacrifice which Jesus Christ makes of Himself on the Cross for His bride, the Church. In this sacrifice there is entirely revealed that plan which God has imprinted on the humanity of man and woman since their creation (cf. Eph 5, 32–33); *the marriage of baptized persons thus becomes a real symbol of that new and eternal covenant sanctioned in the blood of Christ.* The Spirit which the Lord pours forth gives a new heart, and renders man and woman capable of loving one another as Christ has loved us. Conjugal love reaches that fullness to which it is interiorly ordained, conjugal charity, which is *the proper and specific way* in which the spouses participate in and are called to live the very charity of Christ who gave Himself on the Cross. . . . By virtue of the sacramentality of their marriage, spouses are bound to one another in the most profoundly indissoluble manner. *Their belonging to each other is the real representation, by means of the sacramental sign, of the very relationship of Christ with the Church.*[12]

Pope John Paul II concludes his remarks with a summary of what he means when he speaks of sacramental Christian marriage: "In a word it is a question of the normal characteristics of all natural conjugal love, but with a new significance which not only purifies and strengthens them, but raises them to the extent of making them the expression of specifically Christian values."[13]

The Nature of Marital Consent

Marital consent is what brings a marriage into existence, it is the "efficient cause" of the sacrament. Since the promulgation of the 1917 Code of Canon Law, it has been generally appreciated that the older canonical language expressing the right acquired in matrimony as *ius in corpus*, a right to the body of the spouse for the purpose of procreation, has been theologically inadequate for expressing both the procreative *and* the unitive meanings which every conjugal act ought to reflect.[14] Hence, in the new Code we read that "matrimonial consent is an act of the will by which a man and a woman, through an irrevocable covenant, mutually give and accept each other ("sese") in order to establish marriage."[15] This development more clearly reflects the doctrine of Vatican II teaching that marriage

is an institution confirmed by the divine law and receiving its stability, even in the eyes of society, from the human act by which the partners mutually surrender themselves to each other; for the good of the partners, of the children, and of society this sacred bond no longer depends on human decision alone.[16]

This theological and canonical approach to marital consent since Vatican II puts greater stress than formerly on two aspects of it: In the first place, it enhances the notion of consent as an act of *caritas* (charity, love). Those aspects of the marital rights which were formerly seen in the light of justice only—the marital duties, responsibilities and rights—are now seen to be grounded in the *caritas* of the total gift of self. Secondly, the covenantal nature of the "contract" clearly sets matrimony off from other types of contract found in the secular world, puts into clear focus the equality and dignity of the two parties, and reinforces the religious nature of the commitment which is to reflect the qualities of God's covenant with man.

Conjugal Love and Sexual Intercourse

While sexual intimacy is that which specifically differentiates marriage from all other types of friendship, the act of copulation is not enough to make a good natural marriage, much less a sacramental one.

Human sexuality is not merely an external characteristic of a person; rather, it reaches to the depths of "being a person," which is expressed through the body. Human sexuality is something radically different from the sexuality of any other creature. The body's sexuality has meaning given to it by God; since this is so, it is not entirely up to each individual to determine how that sexuality should be expressed. In marriage, the partners become gifts for each other, offering the total gifts of themselves through the unity of their bodies. This is the true expression of masculine and feminine sexuality.

That the sexual expression of conjugal love is intimately tied to the totality of the person is evident in the new Code of Canon Law, which describes a consummated marriage as one where the spouses have performed the conjugal act *humano modo*, that is, in a properly human manner.[17] The mere completion of the sexual act does not constitute true marital consummation; sexual acts accomplished through force or violence do not express the self-gift which marriage is meant by God to be.

We might, at this point, ask ourselves what role acts of sexual intercourse should play in marriage; that is, to what do they contribute? Vatican II teaches that:

Married love is uniquely expressed and perfected by the exercise of the acts proper to marriage. Hence the acts in marriage by which the intimate and chaste union of the spouses takes place are noble and honorable; the truly human performance of these acts fosters the self-giving they signify and enriches the spouses in joy and gratitude. Endorsed by mutual fidelity and, above all, consecrated by Christ's sacrament, this love abides faithfully in mind and body in prosperity and adversity and hence excludes both adultery and divorce.[18]

Thus, *marital* consent, once given, endures and no longer depends solely on human choice. Yet the determination of the partners to maintain their love alive and to make it prosper through various means will always be necessary. Fidelity to a vocation is never automatic.

II. Attitudes to Be Formed Regarding Marriage as a Vocation

In the first section of this Chapter we presented the consciousness at the root of the Church's teachings regarding marriage and the family. In this section, we shall present the attitudes which, in the light of that consciousness, appear to be most deeply related to a Christian view of sexuality.

1) Attitude Toward God and Divine Providence

"Religion" has several meanings, but in its sense as a human virtue it means man's relation to God, and is related to the virtue of justice. God is our Creator, and a religious view of life sees God as our Father. We are the Children of God. Everything we have we have received from Him, and in His provident care He loves us more than we do ourselves:

> That is why I am telling you not to-worry about your life and what you are to eat, nor about your body and how you are to clothe it. Surely life means more than food, and the body more than clothing! . . . So do not worry; do not say, "What are we to eat? What are we to drink? How are we to be clothed?" It is the pagans who set their hearts on all these things. Your heavenly Father knows you need them all. Set your hearts on his kingdom first, and on his righteousness, and all these other things will be given you as well. (Mt 6,25; 31–33)

Pope John Paul II has pointed out that it is through the moral order that God's provident plan is revealed to men:

> Since the moral order reveals and sets forth the plan of God the Creator, for this very reason it cannot be something that harms man, something impersonal. On the contrary, by responding to the deepest demands of the human being created by God, it places itself at the service of that person's full humanity with the delicate and binding love whereby God Himself inspires, sustains and guides every creature towards its happiness.[19]

A sensitivity to morality, a refined conscience formed according to a religious respect for the truth, is the source of man's receptivity toward God's manifesting His will to him, that is, toward "being called by God."

This religious attitude toward life gives the basic meaning and intelligibility to the lives of men and women, and inspires in them a certain humility and charity which, being the virtues most directly opposed to pride ("the inordinate love of self"),[20] capacitates them to incorporate themselves into the plans of God, accepting whatever vocation God wants to give them. Professor Paul Vitz's study[21] documents how it is precisely the desire to justify "inordinate love of self" which is at the root of much "selfist" theory advocating so many of the practices which Christians have traditionally considered simply "wrong."

2) Attitude Toward Sin

Just as the moral order "reveals and sets forth the plan of God the Creator," so infractions of the moral order reveal a person's conscious and free rejection of that plan. There may not be great malice in the person's action; nevertheless, the *evil* remains. Hence, sin is most authentically seen to be "offense to God." It is true that very often the sins people commit also offend others or do damage to themselves; but the same may be said of many actions which people commit, but which are not sins. Seeing sin as primarily offense done to God is part and parcel of a religious view of life which is trying to incorporate itself into the plans of God.

At the same time it is the corrective for a serious confusion between sin and sickness, a confusion pointed out some years ago by a prominent psychologist:

> For several decades we psychologists looked upon the whole matter of sin and moral accountability as a great incubus and acclaimed our liberation from it as epoch-making. But at length we have discovered that to be "free" in this sense, i.e., to have the excuse of being "sick" rather than sinful, is to court the danger of also becoming lost. This danger is, I believe, betokened by the widespread interest in Existentialism which we are presently witnessing. In becoming amoral, ethically neutral, and "free," we have cut the very roots of our being; lost our sense of self-hood and identity; and with neurotics themselves, find ourselves asking: "who *am* I?"[22]

In *Familiaris consortio* Pope John Paul II mentions the special significance of the sacrament of Penance for the strength of spouses and family life:

87

While they discover in faith that sin contradicts not only the covenant with God, but also the covenant between husband and wife and the communion of the family, the married couple and the other members of the family are led to an encounter with God, who is "rich in mercy," who bestows on them His love which is more powerful than sin, and who reconstructs and brings to perfection the marriage covenant and the family communion.[23]

3) Attitude Toward Sex

We have spoken of the Christian view of sexual intimacy whereby such relations in marriage are essentially an expression of the total self-giving which each spouse makes to, and accepts from, the other, thus "imaging" the totally selfless gift of Christ to the Church, and all men. Although the expression of this love in many ways is vital in marriage, still sexual intercourse is the *specific* marital form of doing so; and with the concourse of divine power, children are its natural fruit.

In stark contrast to this view is one which sees sex as "recreational" and whose guiding principle can be stated as "sex in the service of the ego."[24] Even such expressions as "having sex," or "sex object," reveal that such an attitude exists. In viewing sex as an experience enhancing a person's "self-image," those who promote this notion have objectified sex. What is of interest to them is no longer any expression of a gift to the other (since for them, to give "self" is to lose "self"), but rather a deliberate *use* of the other in a way assured to obtain maximum "self"-gratification. Instead of a mutual "imaging" of selfless Love, some psychologists have found that such partners really try to *dominate* the other, and when domination is impossible, to *compete* with the other for the most "self-actualizing" experience.[25]

> Life has become a game where there are only two states: winning and losing; sadist and masochist. . . . Intimate personal relationships become extremely dangerous. If you show weakness, such as a need for love, you get slaughtered; if you withdraw to a machine-like, emotion-free competence and develop complete identification with career you are isolated and starved for intimacy and love. Perhaps there is some relief in temporarily losing the self in sexual or other sensations and afterwards counting each new experience as a score for the self, but a lonely deathlike living is inescapable.[26]

As the author of these words suggests, the only way to avoid this type of development and other humanly negative outcomes is "to stop treat-

88

ing sex as an object, as an experience which men and women take from each other."[27]

In view of the widespread diffusion of the "recreational" view of sex in our society the need stands out more clearly for married people to live and appreciate more fully the virtue of chastity which "is not merely continence, but a decisive affirmation on the part of the will in love. . . . which leads a couple to respect the mystery of sex and ordain it to faithfulness and personal dedication."[28] In the 1981 Apostolic Exhortation on the family, Pope John Paul II reaffirms the beauty and purpose of this virtue which is so important for living any vocation:

> In the Christian view, chastity by no means signifies rejection of human sexuality or lack of esteem for it: rather it signifies spiritual energy capable of defending love from the perils of selfishness and aggressiveness, and able to advance it towards its full realization.[29]

4) Attitudes Toward Family Life

There is always a danger when speaking about marriage to fail to go beyond the specific matters pertaining to that state, and to omit mentioning some of the areas which married people have in common with those who are not married. This is unfortunate, since most of the time any married couple spends together is not taken up in the expression of the mutual love through sexual intercourse. And yet, all the other activities they may do together—the care and education of children, "bringing home the bacon," social and civic duties, etc.—must be equally imbued with the effort to realize their personal vocations from God as partners in marriage. What sorts of preparation or training do spouses need in order to enable them to form an attitude of seeing all these activities in the light of their vocations? Here we can only mention some of the major attitudes which need to be formed in such persons.

First of all, it is very important that they foster their interior lives and those of their children. This will strengthen their sense of discernment in living out their own vocations, in counseling their children wisely, and in making decisions for the common good of the family.[30] They should feel personally the exacting challenge which God has entrusted to them:

> By virtue of their ministry of educating, parents are, through the witness of their lives, the first heralds of the Gospel for their children. Furthermore, by praying with their children, by reading the word of God with them and by introducing

89

them deeply through Christian initiation into the Body of Christ—both the Eucharistic and the ecclesial Body—they become fully parents, in that they are begetters not only of bodily life but also of the life that through the Spirit's renewal flows from the Cross and Resurrection of Christ.

The concrete example and living witness of parents is fundamental and irreplaceable in educating their children to pray. Only by praying together with their children can a father and mother—exercising their royal priesthood—penetrate the innermost depths of their children's hearts and leave an impression that the future events in their lives will not be able to efface.[31]

The Apostolic Exhortation goes on to mention several traditional practices of Christian piety which parents should teach their children to cherish.

The supernatural virtues, including the theological virtues of faith, hope, and charity, come to us with Grace. But they do not facilitate human actions. Rather, they elevate human activity to the supernatural order. Parents—like everyone else—need to acquire the natural, human virtues. *Facility* of action only comes with growth in the "good operative habits"[32] traditionally clustered around the cardinal virtues of prudence, justice, fortitude and temperance. Parents need these human virtues to be able to accomplish *all* their tasks well.

Another attitude which spouses would do well to develop is that of considering their family as the *most* important part of their lives. Someday they will be asked to render an accounting of their parenting to Christ, and so should dedicate all the time that may be necessary to their family life. They must balance all other activities—professional, cultural, recreational, etc.—against the needs of the family. While this may appear at first glance to be a kind of slavery, a deeper consideration of the matter shows that it is really only the day-by-day living out of a free commitment they made at some point in the past. This is a freedom of the sort lived by Jesus who, once He had freely decided to redeem us according to a particular plan, found it necessary to submit Himself to all sorts of limitations. Such a situation is better termed "dedication" than slavery.

Not the least of the tasks of Christian parents is to teach their children to love, not in just any way, but as Christ has loved us. Rooted in the vocation of married couples to participate in God's creative activity is their task to educate, to raise, their children, as *Familiaris consortio* points out very clearly:

The right and duty of parents to give education is essential, since it is connected with the transmission of human life; it is *original and primary* with regard to the educational role of others, on account of the uniqueness of the loving relationship between parents and children; and it is *irreplaceable and inalienable*, and therefore incapable of being entirely delegated to others or usurped by others. In addition to these characteristics, it cannot be forgotten that the most basic element, so basic that it qualifies the educational role of parents, is *parental love*, which finds fulfillment in the task of education as it completes and perfects its service of life: as well as being a *source*, the parents' love is also the animating principle and therefore the *norm* inspiring and guiding all concrete educational activity, enriching it with the values of kindness, constancy, goodness, service, disinterestedness and self-sacrifice that are the most precious fruit of love.[33]

The ultimate reason why the family is the ideal place for children to grow into adulthood rests in the fact that it is the family, united by parental love with the qualities here enumerated by the Holy Father, which provides the proper "environment" for the development of the young human personalities of the children.

It is a tragedy of present-day society that so many children never know the irreplaceable joy of parental love and Christian nurturing in the traditional family unit. It is difficult to contemplate, much less to measure, the irreparable harm that divorce and "alternative life-styles" are doing to our children.

Christian families today, as their counterparts of apostolic times, are called to evangelize a largely unbelieving world,[34] communicating with their lives and with their words the "good news" of a family formed many years ago which was not merely a symbol of the love of God, but the very occasion wherein "the Word was made flesh" (Jn 1, 14), wherein God gave Himself totally to the human race (cf. Phil 2, 5–8), in order to bring us all Home: "Oh God, who hast deigned to give us the shining example of the Holy Family; mercifully grant us that, by imitating their domestic virtues in the bond of charity, we may enjoy eternal rewards in the joy of Thy Home."[35]

Discussion Questions

1. What is the main difference between the reproduction of any other living species, and human procreation?

91

2. What reason can be given for saying that a child is a "gift"? From whom is it a gift? To whom?
3. What is the "sign" of the sacrament of Matrimony? Should Christian spouses be guided by this sign in showing love for one another?
4. What is the Christian vocation to marriage and the family? Do you think that fidelity to that vocation is "automatic," or does it require some effort on everyone's part? What ideals of the love required by Christian marriage does the Church hold out for married couples to imitate?
5. The quest for sanctity in marriage requires that spouses live many virtues and that they teach their children to live them also. List as many of these virtues as you can, and show why they are important. [*Hint:* the Apostolic Exhortation *Familiaris Consortio* mentions many such virtues, especially in Part III.]

Notes

1. Cf. Paul C. Vitz, *Psychology As Religion: The Cult of Self-Worship* (Grand Rapids, MI: Eerdmans 1977) for a brief, penetrating critique of these "assaults." Additional works of interest include: C. S. Lewis, *God in the Dock* (Grand Rapids, MI: Eerdmans 1970); Ludwig von Bertalanffy, *Robots, Men and Minds* (New York: Braziller 1967); Ernest Becker, *Escape from Evil* (New York: Free Press 1975) and *Denial of Death* (New York: Free Press 1973; Paul Zweig, *The Heresy of Self-Love* (Princeton, NJ: Princeton University Press 1980). Additional bibliography may be found in Vitz, *op. cit.*, pp. 136–144. Vitz signals one of the reasons why scientists have begun to react against "faddish" selfist theory, on p. 62: "That much of selfism is dependent on a broad base of economic prosperity has been driven home in the last few years by inflation and recession. It has become very hard to actualize oneself at today's prices."

2. Karol Wojtyla/Pope John Paul II, *Sources of Renewal: The Implementation of Vatican II* (San Francisco: Harper and Row 1980) 437 pp.

3. *Ibid.*, pp. 15–18; 203–206.

4. Edward O. Wilson, *Sociobiology: The New Synthesis* (Cambridge, MA: Harvard University Press 1975) p. 315.

5. St. Thomas Aquinas, *Summa Theologiae*, I, q. 45, a.5.

6. J. Escriva de Balaguer, *Christ Is Passing By* (Chicago: Scepter Press 1974) #27. Msgr. Escriva, who died in 1975, founded the personal Prelature Opus Dei in 1928. He wrote and preached that marriage was a vocation from at least the early '30s.

7. Cf. Rom 8, 14–30; Pastoral Constitution on the Church in the Modern World *(Gaudium et spes)*, #22; John Paul II, Encyclical *Redemptor hominis*, #8.

8. *Redemptor hominis*, #13.

9. J. Escriva de Balaguer, *op. cit.*, #23.

10. Dogmatic Constitution on the Church *(Lumen gentium)*, #11.

11. Dz 970; translation from *The Church Teaches* (St. Louis: B. Herder 1955) p. 336.

12. John Paul II, Apostolic Exhortation on the Role of the Christian Family in the Modern World *(Familiaris consortio)*, #13 [Emphasis added.]

13. *Ibid.*

14. Paul VI, Encyclical *Humanae vitae*, #12.

15. Canon 1057, 2. Translation from *Codex Iuris Canonici* (Roma: Libreria Editrice Vaticana 1983) Canon Law Society of America, 1983. [Emphasis added.]

16. *Gaudium et spes*, #48.

17. Canon 1061, 1. Translation from *loc. cit.*

18. *Gaudium et spes*, #49.

19. *Familiaris consortio*, #34.

20. St. Thomas Aquinas, *op. cit.*, II–II, q. 162.

21. Cf. Paul C. Vitz, *op. cit.*, in Note 1.

22. O. Hobart Mowrer, "Sin, the lesser of two evils," *American Psychologist* XV (1960) pp. 302–304.

23. *Familiaris consortio*, #58.

24. Paul C. Vitz, *op. cit.*, p. 34; cf. John Money, "Recreational and procreational sex," *New York Times*, September 13, 1975, p. 23.

25. Cf. Herbert Hendin, *The Age of Sensation* (New York: Norton 1975), and the discussion of his findings in Vitz, *op. cit.*, pp. 120–126.

26. Paul C. Vitz, *op. cit.*, p. 125.

27. *Ibid.*, p. 123.

28. J. Escriva de Balaguer, *op. cit.*, #25.

29. *Familiaris consortio*, #33.

30. *Ibid.*, #5, 36–41, 49–50, 66.

31. *Ibid.*, #39 & 60.

32. St. Thomas Aquinas, *op. cit.*, I–II, q.55.

33. *Familiaris consortio*, #36. [Emphasis in the original.]

34. *Ibid.*, #49–64.

35. Prayer from the Feast of the Holy Family, *Breviarium Romanum*, Vol. I (translated from the Latin).

Preview of
Chapter Eight

● This chapter could not have been written twenty years ago—it discusses natural family planning as realistic, reliable, and even enriching within marriage.

● Perhaps the strongest asset of natural family planning springs from its inherent mutuality.

● The best motive for adopting natural family planning is love— preserving and reverencing the authentic act of conjugal love, marital intercourse.

● Contraception removes from the conjugal act its inherent orientation to express totally unselfish love in imitation of Christ's total self-giving to the Church.

● Pope John Paul II summed up the challenge facing the natural family planning movement as twofold: instilling conviction and offering pastoral help.

CHAPTER 8

Natural Family Planning As Enriching Marriages

This chapter could not have been written twenty years ago. It will discuss natural family planning as now understood, not only as a realistic approach to responsible parenthood, but as a practice enriching and deepening marital relationships. This appreciation of natural family planning is dawning on married couples all over the world with the brightness and brilliance of an April sunrise. *This new dawn follows the darkness and gloom of the worldwide birth control controversy.*

In this twentieth century modern health care marvelously reduced infant mortality. Women's fertility began returning promptly after delivery of each new baby because of improved diet and because breast feeding was replaced by bottle-feeding. Couples who have four and five babies in the first half-dozen years of marriage face tremendous financial and emotional strain in urban societies.

The rallying call for "planned parenthood" generated popular sympathy. But the early contraceptives created a genuine barrier to satisfactory marital intercourse, because either the husband wore a condom or the wife inserted a diaphragm. Up to the historic acceptance of the principle of marital contraception by the Lambeth Conference of the Anglican Communion in 1930, no Christian denomination had approved contraception.

The practice of couples spacing children by recording their monthly period of fertility got underway in the 1930's. Two physician researchers, Drs. Ogino in Japan and Knaus in Austria, had independently discovered that a woman's ovulation occurs in a limited period in the middle of the menstrual cycle. Couples could now estimate their fertile period on the basis of calendar records of the longest and shortest menstrual periods of the wife.

While calendar rhythm was 100% reliable for some couples, especially those where the wife had very regularly occurring menstrual cycles, it was unreliable for at least 10% to 20% of couples, enough to generate considerable scepticism. But condoms and diaphragms were only about 90% effective in actual use. Massive research continued until the birth control pills appeared in the late 1950's. Now the health risks of the pill have made surgical sterilization an increasingly common approach to birth control.

Scientific Natural Family Planning

However, in the 25 years following the Ogino and Knaus breakthrough in 1930, *more scientific research on signs and symptoms of fertility led to scientific natural family planning.* Couples now may accurately document, through daily temperature records of the wife, the fact that the fertile period of their monthly cycle has ended. Women who learn to observe the monthly appearance at the opening of the vagina of a mucus discharge can anticipate when their fertile period will occur. They can also learn to notice changes in the cervix which coincide with fertility.

In 1971, a national organization called the Couple to Couple League was formed by John and Sheila Kippley and Dr. Konald Prem in St. Paul, Minnesota, to train and certify couples teaching natural family planning. They follow the Sympto-Thermal Method (STM) which teaches couples to keep temperature records as well as observe mucus and cervical signs of fertility. They have certified over 600 teaching couples in 47 states of the U.S. and six foreign countries.

The Ovulation Method (OM) of natural family planning relies exclusively on the woman's mucus discharge at the opening of the vagina as a sign of fertility. Doctors John and Lynn Billings of Australia have popularized this method internationally and work with the federation called World Organization, Ovulation Method—Billings (WOOMB). Dr. Thomas Hilgers of the Creighton University School of Medicine in Omaha, Nebraska, has established a program of OM training for natural family planning practitioners (NFPP) as teachers of natural family planning, and a second stage program preparing natural family planning educators (NFPE) for teacher training.

The blossoming of such programs in natural family planning today all over the United States *indicates a trend which may well expand vastly before the turn of the century.* It offers a solution to the birth control challenge far more in accord with the Judeo-Christian tradition of sexual morality than the approach adopted by organizations like the Planned Parenthood Federation.

Such organizations as the latter have fostered a view of sexual activity as recreational rather than procreational. Their attitude to an unplanned pregnancy as a contraceptive failure readily tolerates abortion as a contraceptive back-up. Their enthusiasm for using contraceptive protection against an unwanted pregnancy readily condones sexual intercourse by unmarried persons. It supports the anti-child bias of population alarmists who would classify pregnancy as a disease.

The natural family planning organizations, on the other hand, teach profound respect of human fertility as a unique gift. In their eyes a surprise pregnancy means an unexpected gift of new life rather than an occasion for abortion. Their values are rooted in respect for life and the life-process whereas the values of contraceptive organizations are rooted in the manipulation and suppression of the life-process.

Assets and Effectiveness of NFP

Perhaps the strongest asset of natural family planning springs from its inherent mutuality: Neither spouse can use the method alone, whereas they do use contraceptives alone. The interpersonal significance of conjugal intercourse seems to demand an interpersonal involvement in family planning rather than a solitary effort. One might even argue that psychological as well as physiological risks spring from the single-spouse practice of contraception or sterilization in marriage.

Couples who mutually assume responsibility for family planning share a common sequence of "courtship" and "honeymoon" periods in their marital life. Instead of relegating their fertility to medical, mechanical, or surgical suppression, they maintain a continual awareness of their life power as a gift and a responsibility. The periods of abstinence from conjugal intercourse which last about ten days per month challenge them to communicate their love in words and signs they might otherwise neglect.

Teachers of natural family planning report that couples need time to learn the method and become relaxed with it. *But, soon after they begin using it, many couples report subtle changes in their relationship with each other.* They notice they are becoming more generous with each other, more unselfish about each other's preferences, and more openly expressive of their love, as in courtship days.

These clear assets of natural family planning all relate to the mutuality of the spouses. They will not occur in cases where one spouse resists use of the method or where both spouses use the method for selfish reasons or even combine it with barrier contraceptives during fertile times. These situations indicate real problems in the marriage which need to be resolved, perhaps through spiritual efforts of prayer and sacrifice.

Proponents of natural family planning readily note that this method facilitates planning pregnancies as well as avoiding surprise pregnancies. Often 10% or more of the couples learning the method do so initially to increase their prospects of parenthood. The emphasis on understanding exactly when conjugal relations are fertile is completely ignored by the practice of contraception which focuses only on suppressing fertility.

Statistics on the effectiveness of all forms of family planning need careful interpretation. Proponents of the Sympto-Thermal Method of natural family planning were pleased by a U.S. Department of Health and Human Services leaflet published in 1980. It announced that government research showed NFP to be 98% effective.[1] The so-called user-effectiveness will vary, however, depending on whether the persons using the method are seeking simply to space births or to limit all further births.

The Couple to Couple League has reports of only 156 unplanned pregnancies after ten years in which they have instructed 44,000 couples. If that were a complete total of surprise pregnancies, the actual user-effectiveness of STM would be 99.7%. Even if the number of surprises were 10 times that number the effectiveness would still be 97%, which is comparable to the user-effectiveness of the birth control pill and more effective than other contraceptives.

Obviously, user-effectiveness represents the practical goal of family planning. Teachers of scientific natural family planning are universally agreed that *it rivals artificial methods in user-effectiveness when couples are properly instructed and motivated.*

Love as a Motive for NFP

The motives which commonly prompt the use of natural family planning today include a widespread fear of the medical after-effects of contraceptive pills and a distaste for barrier methods as clumsy and displeasing. Yet the religious tradition which opposes contraceptives relies on a very positive motive. *It teaches that natural family planning preserves the authenticity of conjugal intercourse as an act of love,* whereas contraception undermines the significance of the conjugal act of love, in a certain sense, trivializing it.

Chapter One of this volume began with a consideration of love as the central vocation which Christianity proclaims for all people of all time. Sexual intercourse can be described as the unique expression of marital love. The book of *Genesis* portrayed both the unique and intimate unity of sexual intercourse and the unique gift of fruitfulness or procreativity.

"Precisely because the love of husband and wife is a unique participation in the mystery of life and of the love of God Himself," wrote Pope John Paul II recently, "the Church knows that she has received the special mission of guarding and protecting the lofty dignity of marriage and the most serious responsibility of the transmission of human life."[2]

The act of conjugal love or marital intercourse hence must be examined and respected in its unique power as a sign among all possible signs of love which carry out the general Christian vocation of love. The Biblical term for this general love to which Christians are called is the Greek word, *agape.* It describes God's own infinite love within the Trinity which Jesus brought into human lives. "As the Father has loved me," Jesus said, "so have I loved you, live on in my love." (Jn. 15:9) He added, "Love one another as I have loved you." (Jn. 15:12) In Chapter One this was described as "The New Testament Law of Love:"

God wanted to create beings who would be eternally united with Him in His love. Jean Guitton described this love as a "sweet and burning, motionless and endlessly progressive state of life." The religious term for this love is *agapeic love,* and the first epistle of John declares, "God is love (*agape*)." (1 Jn. 4:8)

The Christian life of agapeic love cannot be expressed exclusively toward God, for "One who has no love for the brother he has seen cannot love the God he has not seen." (1 Jn. 4:20) The key to agapeic love is selfless giving, "The way we came to understand love was that He laid down His life for us, we too must lay down our lives for our brothers." (1 Jn. 3:16) In Christian life all human actions should flow from the abiding presence of the Spirit and should manifest selfless concern for others rooted in agapeic love or charity.

In the case of conjugal love, this doctrine means that the actions of spouses directed toward one another should manifest their interior holiness and love. These actions may be touches, kisses, acts of service and concern, verbal communication, or the unique act of conjugal love, marital intercourse. *Since spouses are called to love each other as Christ loves the Church, all expressions of conjugal love are clearly meant to express agapeic love.*

Contraception and Authentic Conjugal Love

The Second Vatican Council described Christian conjugal love when it wrote, "Authentic married love is caught up into divine love and is directed and enriched by the redemptive power of Christ and the salvific action of the Church.[3] Church teaching insists that married love must be *"authentic."* What does this require?

First of all, the couple must have entered a marital covenant. A covenant is a bond in which two persons give themselves to each other. In the marriage covenant husband and wife have given themselves totally, exclusively and indissolubly to each other. The act of marital intercourse will be "inauthentic" without that mutual giving of self: non-convenanted intercourse cannot be *authentic* marital intercourse.

Is anything else required for *"authentic"* conjugal intercourse? Pope Paul VI specified two further conditions in his famous encyclical, *Humanae Vitae*. First, the act must be a true act of love, not one "imposed upon a partner without regard for his or her condition and lawful desires."[4] Secondly, the reciprocal act of love must not jeopardize the "responsibility to transmit life which God the Creator, according to particular laws, inserted therein." The Pope teaches that the spouses must not eliminate their openness to life by contraception or sterilization which destroy the meaning and finality of their act of conjugal intercourse.[5]

Catholic doctrine, then, holds that in each and every act of conjugal intercourse the couple are affirming and celebrating the fact that God has made them male and female and has given them to each other. They cannot love one another *authentically* without the two conditions Paul VI outlined. Whenever a couple intervene to eliminate the procreative meaning of their conjugal act they cause it to be *"inauthentic."* It no longer truly expresses their covenant gift to each other because they

100

have destroyed the capacity of their act to generate life through love. Their act of giving has been compromised by withholding.

Furthermore, *this intervention removes the act's inherent orientation to express totally unselfish, that is, agapeic, love in imitation of Christ's total self-giving to the Church.* Subjectively, the spouses may intend to express genuinely agapeic love, but they have removed the true agapeic character from their conjugal act.

Pope John Paul II described this impact of contraception in one powerful sentence: "Thus the innate language that expresses the total reciprocal self-giving of husband and wife is overlaid, through contraception, by an objectively contradictory language, namely, that of not giving oneself totally to the other."[6]

Couples who practice natural family planning rather than contraception in order to preserve the authenticity of their conjugal acts have a strong and solid motive for their decision. They avoid ever contradicting the language of their love. Their rejection of contraception itself speaks a language of respect for their sacred privilege of transmitting life through procreation.

The Contraceptive Mentality and NFP

The so-called contraceptive mentality which appeared in recent decades divorces the vocation to parenthood from marriage. It supposes that couples may treat their procreative gift as a mere optional accessory to marriage, an option to be chosen purely on the basis of sufficient mutual inclination toward parenthood.

The profound teaching on marriage at the Second Vatican Council left no room for this mentality. It said forthrightly, "Married couples should regard it as their proper mission to transmit human life and to educate their children."[7]

A couple could choose to practice natural family planning as a selfish escape from parenthood. This would become an actual manifestation of the contraceptive mentality. Pope Paul VI described responsible parenthood in a way which opposes this mentality: "Responsible parenthood is exercised, either by the deliberate and generous decision to raise a numerous family, or by the decision, made for grave motives and with due respect for the moral law, to avoid for the time being, or even for an indeterminate period, a new birth."[8]

Chapter Twelve will review some instances where a couple may feel the risk of genetic defect forces them to forego procreation entirely. However, even here, couples must beware of looking on children exclusively as a burden, a drain on parental energies, an economic liability, or an invasion of marital privacy.

The Second Vatican Council reminded couples that children "greatly contribute to the good of the parents themselves" and that "children as living members of the family contribute in their own way to the sanctification of their parents."[9] Couples unable to bear children suffer a genuine privation, but "marriage still retains its character of being a whole manner and communion of life and preserves its value and indissolubility."[10]

Marriage Enrichment Through NFP

Teachers of natural family planning respect parenthood as a privilege to be undertaken joyfully and generously. Perhaps this partially explains why the positive enrichment of marriage relationships is becoming more and more obvious among those who practice natural family planning for the good of their families.

John and Sheila Kippley, pioneers of natural family planning, have been impressed from the beginning by the positive benefits it brings to the marriage relationship. "In the very first class we taught back in 1971," they write, "we had couples coming off the pill. They came to us after a couple months and shared with us that they had noticed a distinct improvement in their personal marriage relationships since starting NFP. *That experience has become commonplace.*

"We started out apologizing for the normal abstinence. Now we know that the abstinence is an asset, not a liability in actual practice. That's not to say it's necessarily easy. It's very much like the totality of the Christian faith: It's not necessarily easy, but it's the greatest asset any one of us can have."

What the Kippleys and others have learned can be summarized in terms of agapeic love. When a Christian couple seek to model their covenant on Christ's covenant with the Church, their call to agapeic love becomes a vivid and almost overwhelming challenge. The sacrifice of some occasions of marital intercourse becomes another sign of their self-giving to each other. It prepares them for a deeper love and a love which can both transcend and transform their actions of marital intercourse.

One would expect, on the other hand, that the practice of *contraception would weaken the marriage bond because it removes the objective agapeic meaning from marital intercourse.* Adequate data is not yet available to document this, but the spiraling divorce ratio gives no indication that the

102

widespread practice of contraception is strengthening marriage as its proponents have alleged it would.

The Future

When the Second Vatican Council ended in 1965, the developments of the next two decades were not foreseen. In these years the contraceptive pill has produced massive disenchantment, sterilization has taken on near epidemic proportions in the United States, and natural family planning has gained new credibility and a beginning ground swell of support from enthusiastic couples.

One veteran teacher of natural family planning recently listed three wishes for the future of natural family planning instruction:

1) That spiritual, medical, psychological, and family counselors would realize the importance and benefits of NFP and refer couples for competent instruction in it.
2) That hospitals, dioceses, and parishes sponsor the training of NFP teachers and promote their work through their own organizational structures.
3) That there be a more positive cooperation between persons teaching natural family planning according to the various methods, such as STM and OM.

All three of these wishes are among the objectives of a "Diocesan Plan for Natural Family Planning Development" sponsored by the National Conference of Catholic Bishops under the direction of their Committee for Prolife Activities.[11] A key to the success of such efforts of the future will be found in quality control of teacher training and extensive promotional efforts to convey the actual method of successful natural family planning and the motivational background described in this chapter.

Pope John Paul II summed up the Church's mission in natural family planning when he wrote, "The ecclesial community at this time must take on the task *of instilling conviction* and *offering pastoral help* to those who wish to live out their parenthood in a truly responsible way."[12]

Discussion Questions

1. Can you outline the modern development of natural family planning since 1930?

2. What is the strongest asset of natural family planning? Why?
3. Can you describe the two chief methods of natural family planning, STM and OM?
4. How can you explain love as a primary motive for natural family planning?
5. Can the decision to postpone marital intercourse be an expression of agapeic love?
6. How could you describe the contraceptive mentality?
7. What paradox can you find in the enrichment of marriage relationships through natural family planning? How can you explain this paradox?

Notes

1. "Natural Family Planning," U.S. Department of Health and Human Services, publication no. (HSA) 80–5621.

2. *The Apostolic Exhortation on the Family (Familiaris Consortio)*, Nov. 22, 1981, Vatican Text, #29.

3. *The Church in the Modern World (Gaudium et Spec)*, in *Vatican Council II, The Conciliar and Post Conciliar Documents*, ed. by Austin Flannery O.P. (Collegeville, MN: The Liturgical Press, 1975), #48.

4. *Of Human Life (Humanae Vitae)*, July 29, 1968, (Huntington, IN: Our Sunday Visitor Inc., 1968), #13.

5. *Ibid.*

6. *The Apostolic Exhortation on the Family*, #32.

7. *The Church in the Modern World*, #50.

8. *Of Human Life*, #10.

9. *The Church in the Modern World*, #50, #48.

10. *Ibid.* #50.

11. Program directed by Rev. Msgr. James T. McHugh, 1511 K St. N.W., Room 333, Washington, D.C. 20005.

12. *The Apostolic Exhortation on the Family*, #35.

PART TWO

Specific Sexual Issues

Preview of
Chapter Nine

- Contraceptives have been widely adopted because of their effectiveness in preventing pregnancy. In actual use their effectiveness is always less than their theoretical effectiveness.

- The IUD and, in some instances the contraceptive pills, do not prevent conception, they cause the fertilized egg to perish.

- The alleged safety of all contraceptive methods is contradicted by abundant research data; the perfect contraceptive has not yet been found.

- It seems that artificial contraception and greater moral permissiveness have interacted with and promoted each other in contemporary America.

- Social research shows various attitudinal reasons why couples choose smaller families and contraception. It does not show conclusively whether the availability of contraception acts as a primary stimulus to increasing sexual permissiveness.

CHAPTER 9

Contraception and Sterilization for Birth Control

What has motivated our contemporary society to adopt artificial contraception, including contraceptive sterilization, as a significant part of its "life-style"? The answer is clearly *effectiveness*. Artificial contraception has been seen and accepted as an *effective* way of achieving certain goals and at the same time avoiding certain problems.

There is no doubt that artificial means of contraception are effective.[1] It is clear, however, that *the effectiveness of some of these means has been exaggerated*, while *some negative side effects have been played down or ignored*. It is obvious, for instance, that however effective the pill is in avoiding pregnancy, its widespread use is also an open invitation to the venereal disease epidemics which we have experienced in recent years. Whatever protection the condom offered in this regard, the pill obviously did not. Yet, when the pill first began to be touted as a major "answer" to our fertility problems, little if any attention was paid to this aspect of its use.

107

Persons who oppose artificial contraception on moral grounds must be careful not to fall into the trap of exaggerating the bad effects which this practice has on human lives spiritually, physically, psychologically, and sociologically. Nor must they exaggerate the effectiveness or overlook the limitations of natural family planning.

Apparent Effectiveness of Various Types of Artificial Contraception

It is not accurate to speak *simply* of the effectiveness of artificial means of contraception for *avoiding* pregnancy. As we shall note later, some of these means do not prevent a pregnancy, but rather *bring one to an early halt through an unnoticed abortion.*

"The pill" is actually a name used to cover three pills, each of different composition or strength. The *regular* pill is a combination of two man-made hormones, estrogen and progestrogen. There are about 30 brands on the market, and each has a slightly different amount of these two synthetic chemicals. Governments in various parts of the world have moved to reduce the hormonal level of these "regular" pills. Still, *if taken as directed,* they are considered 99.5% effective.[2]

The second type is the "low dose" pill. Precisely because they have a lesser quantity of the two synthetic hormones than the "regular" pill, they may be slightly less effective.

The third type, the "mini-pill," has only one hormone, progestrogen. It must be taken every day *at approximately the same hour.* Forgetting to take it on time destroys its effectiveness, though when used as directed it is considered 97% effective.

The intra-uterine device (IUD) is a coil or loop inserted into the uterus. It comes in two types, one of them considered more suitable for women who have already given birth. They are reported to be between 94% and 99% effective.

Diaphragms, when properly fitted over the cervix and used with a spermicidal foam, jelly, or pessary, are considered up to 95% effective. However, incorrect positioning of the diaphragm and the varying effectiveness of the spermicides used mean that total effectiveness may be closer to 80%.

A condom of high quality is 95% effective when used properly. Seminal fluid can easily escape, however, through careless use or accident, and thus the condom's true effectiveness is about 80%.

Withdrawal of the penis and ejaculation away from the vaginal area may be 70% to 80% effective. One main reason for failure is that healthy sperm are often released within the vagina *before* ejaculation occurs.

The controversial drug Depo-Provera is taken by injection every three months or by implantation under the skin for a year at a time. The injections are about 99% effective. Studies on the effectiveness of the skin implants are not yet complete.[3]

Female sterilization is by hysterectomy or by tubal ligation, cauterization, or clamping. Male sterilization is by vasectomy. Surgical sterilization of males and females is almost 100% effective, although males may continue to release sperm for as long as three months after the operation.[4]

Contraception: Real or Only Apparent?

Some of the techniques described above, *within the limits of their effectiveness*, truly *prevent* conception. This is true of the diaphragm, the condom, and withdrawal. *Other techniques, however, may also allow for conception to occur, and then the fertilized egg to perish.* This seems to be true of the IUD.[5]

Though all the evidence is not yet in, this *may* also be the case with the contraceptive pills, all of which disrupt the normal growth pattern of the lining of the womb.[6] The "low dose" and "mini-pill" seem to have to rely even more on this latter effect than the "regular" pill does. It is not at all clear, then, that these pills always or even often succeed in actually *preventing* a conception by stopping ovulation or inhibiting the sperm as they are supposed to.[7] If it were proven, then, that the pills do not inhibit ovulation, we would have to conclude that such pills often abort newly conceived life by depriving it of the womb environment in which alone it will have an opportunity to survive.

Because contraceptive injections also disrupt the lining of the womb, the same doubts must presently prevail.[8] It is not yet clear whether or not the skin-implant chemicals act in this way.

Female sterilization through tubal ligation may also create an abortive situation. For the ectopic pregnancy rate after tubal ligation is 20 times the normal rate.[9] Sperm may pass up through an incompletely closed tube and reach and fertilize an ovum, thus creating a new living individual. This embryonic human being, however, being so much larger than the sperm, cannot pass back down through whatever small opening there may be in the tube, will lodge in the tube above the point of ligation, and eventually perish. Such a tubal pregnancy involves also, of course, great danger to the woman. This brings us to another serious drawback with many forms of artificial contraception for the woman or man who makes use of them: their safety.

109

Is Artificial Contraception Safe?

As was indicated in the early part of this chapter, one of the most popular forms of artificial contraception, when combined with the sexual promiscuity so widely accepted in our time, invites epidemics of venereal disease. The recent outbreak of herpes made news precisely for this reason. It is turning out, then, that such is going to be the case with a number of the above mentioned new technological contraceptive arrangements which *allow nonetheless for "safe" flesh-to-flesh contact in sexually active persons*. Needless to say, venereal disease can thus easily be passed also to an innocent husband, wife, or fetal child.

Venereal disease, however, is not the only concern. A number of the "advanced" methods have been advanced only by hastily passing over other possible detrimental effects to human health that they might pose. While such detrimental effects must not be imagined or exaggerated, neither can the evidence for them be ignored.

The Pill: Safe?

A 1978 study on the pill estimated that women who *take the pill*, are over *30*, and *smoke* are *4 to 8 times more likely to die* of a blood clot than are non-users of the pill.[10]

The same study claims that the risk of heart attack for women in this category is almost 3 times higher than for those who do not use the pill. If, in *addition* to being over 35 and a smoker, the woman has *high blood pressure*, or smokes *more than 15 cigarettes* a day, or has *high blood fat levels*, or has *diabetes*, then any two of these additional factors could increase the risk of heart attack *128-fold*.

Five to eight percent of women will develop mild to severe blood pressure problems as a result of using the pill. *Strokes* resulting from the rise in blood pressure are estimated to be 9.5 *times more frequent* in pill users than in non-users. While not always fatal, especially in a younger woman, such a stroke nonetheless has a devastating effect on her and her family as she must struggle for months to overcome the resulting physical or mental impairment.

A recent study by the United States Center for Disease Control in Atlanta, Georgia, reports that a serious type of liver tumor has been showing up in women, most often in those who have been on the pill for 7 or more years.[11]

In addition to these and a number of other health problems for the woman herself, certain birth defects and poor quality and quantity of breast milk also are at risk for pill users.[12] From time to time over the past few years reports have surfaced of other possible problems, but also of some advantageous side-effects. All of this makes it obvious that we have yet much to learn about all that these pills do to a woman's body.

The IUD: Safe?

The IUD, especially during its first year of use, is subject to spontaneous expulsion by the uterus.[13] Five percent of such expulsions are not noticed by the woman, and leave her liable to impregnation. Certain types of IUD tend to pierce the uterine wall and move into the tissues of surrounding organs, where they may embed themselves.[14]

Infections of the pelvis are estimated to be 3 to 5 times more likely for IUD users.[15] Recent studies indicate that such infection may damage the fallopian tubes, sometimes seriously enough to cause sterility.

Moreover, 4% to 6% of IUD users become pregnant in spite of the device; 30% to 50% of such pregnancies will miscarry.[16] The likelihood of such miscarriage is greatly reduced, however, if the IUD is removed during the first trimester, the earlier the better. Five to ten percent of such pregnancies in IUD users are ectopic, with the tube usually rupturing at 8 to 12 weeks and very often having to be removed later.

Women who have never had a child often experience severe pain and damage to the cervix as the IUD is inserted. Menstrual disorders, cramps, and backaches are common complaints.

Male Contraceptive Practices: Safe?

The condom cannot be used without lubricating chemicals which tend to irritate the delicate lining of the vagina.[17] The practice of withdrawal during intercourse often causes constant anxiety during sexual union for fear that the man will not withdraw in time. Over a long period of time the practice may lead to premature ejaculation on the part of the man, and to failure to achieve orgasm on the part of the woman.

Contraceptive Injections and Implants: Safe?

It *seems* that Depo-Provera may cause a number of problems. For this reason, the U.S. Food and Drug Administration will not allow its use within the United States for contraception. *"Its benefits for this purpose to patients in the United States do not justify the risk."*[18] The Australian govern-

111

ment has banned its use without special permission. Nevertheless, American firms are exporting Depo-Provera to Third-World countries, and many population-control groups are promoting it outside the U.S.A.

The risks of which the F.D.A. report speaks include the following: Progressive decline and even permanent termination of bleeding with each cycle; unpredictable and excessive bleeding; probable destruction of the normal growth of the lining of the uterus; long delay or even termination of fertility once Depo-Provera is withdrawn; congenital malformation of a fetus should an unwanted pregnancy occur; poor breast milk; headaches; depression; loss of sexual energy; and pains in the limbs.

Skin implants are suspected of many of these same health hazards. In addition, there are often infections at the site of implant.

Tubal Ligation and Hysterectomy: Safe?

Tubal ligations are often complicated by severe bleeding, pelvic infection, and, as we have noted, ectopic pregnancies, which are 20 times more common in sterilized women than in other women.[19] Moreover, the fallopian tubes carry blood vessels to the uterus, and ligation cuts down the normal supply of blood to the organ. This may later necessitate a hysterectomy.

As is well known, hysterectomy frequently leads to depression and sexual dysfunction. Subsequent psychiatric referral is 3 times more common with hysterectomy than with other operations. One study shows that one third of women who have had such surgery report deterioration of their sexual relationships as a result of the operation.

Male Sterilization: Safe?

Infection and hemorrhage are immediate problems in many vasectomies. Recent research indicates also that sperm which are not ejaculated break down.[20] The particles of the sperm then pass into the blood stream, where *antibodies are produced to fight them.* It is now suspected that thyroid and joint disorders, heart and circulatory diseases, and diabetes result from this reaction. In addition, some men feel that they are not whole after the operation, and severe anxiety and loss of self-esteem result. A physician expert in this field remarked a few years ago:

Vasectomy seems to be a very simple operation, but people have been taking too limited and short-term a view of it. The body does not like being attacked, even in simple ways surgically, and can pay you back in a most roundabout fashion.[21]

Happy with Artificial Contraception?

The above data make it evident that *we are far from having a perfect contraceptive, quite apart from the moral viewpoint.* Studies indicate that many people sooner or later face up to this fact, for *significant numbers discontinue the various contraceptive paths on which they have embarked.*[22]

In Australia, 51% of women on the pill discontinued it within one year; 30% did so in England. Thirty percent have the IUD removed within a year. Within the same period, 78% of the couples who use the condom abandon that method, and 44% of women on Depo-Provera stop using it. Sixty-five percent of couples who use the diaphragm and spermicide combination discontinue it within 6 months. It is not so easy, of course, to abandon a tubal ligation or vasectomy once it has been done, but increasing numbers of people seek to have the operations reversed. At this point, however, repairs of tubal ligations are successful only 50% of the time, and repairs of vasectomies even less so.

Has Artificial Contraception Changed Our Thinking?

Artificial contraception, including contraceptive sterilization, has obvious effects, some considered desirable and others not considered so, on the bodies of human beings.

Has artificial contraception caused a change in our society and the way of thinking of our people?

One change is certain: The United States birth rate has dropped dramatically.[23] But has artificial contraception *caused* this drop? And has the widespread availability and acceptance of artificial contraception also caused a rise in abortion, in pre-marital sexuality, and in couples' living together without marriage? Or is it the other way around, have these contemporary phenomena been the causes of the availability and acceptance of artificial contraception? *Is there a third alternative? Have artificial contraception and greater moral permissiveness interacted with, and promoted each other?*

What evidence is available—and it is by no means exhaustive—indicates that the third alternative points to the truth. Sociological studies suggest that artificial contraception is not *simply* the cause or the effect of the decline in births or rise in sexual permissiveness. It is *both* a cause *and* an effect.

It should be emphasized that studies of the statistical relationship between artificial contraception and what many would consider a deterioration of moral life in society are by no means adequate by sociological standards. One representative sociologist insists that only a concentrated study of many *individual* families over 25 or 30 years can enable us even to begin to predict how the attitudes and life-styles of other similar families will work themselves out.[24]

Moreover, most of the studies which have been done on contraceptive behavior have been criticized for being unclear in the definitions of what they are looking for, inadequate in the procedures they followed, and inconsistent in the interpretation of their results.

Does Artificial Contraception Lead to Smaller Families—or Vice-Versa?

Despite such problems, certain conclusions seem clear:

1) There is a dramatically more widespread use of artificial contraception both inside and outside of marriage today then ever before in American history.
2) There has been a radical change among Catholics on this issue.[25]
3) Couples who are more traditional, that is, both more stable in the husband-wife relationship, and supported by an "extended family" of grandparents, aunts and uncles, and the like, have more children than couples whose union is unstable and isolated from relatives.[26]
4) No *one* factor, such as the availability and acceptance of contraception, leads to a lower birth rate.[27]

Some other social research projects, while needing careful scrutiny and more supplemental work, have come to some thought-provoking conclusions.

1) Any particular religious affiliation is *at present* not obviously characteristic either of those who chose to have only a small family, or of those who have recourse to artificial contraception. *Exactly what the present impact of religious belief is in this area is most difficult to assess.*[28]

2) The married couples representative of a generation which accepts artificial contraception and abortion are a "new breed" who *cannot be*

114

expected to have the same kind of parent-child relationship to which our society was formerly accustomed.[29]

3) *"Buying into" contemporary life-styles and spending patterns* is the single most typical characteristic of couples who drastically limit the size of their families. This is especially true of couples where the woman has a college education or more. For her, education often means postponement of marriage until she has completed her academic work. It also means a number of years of working to make profitable use of her education. Finally, it generally means that she expects to enjoy a high standard of living. These expectations are hard to meet if one has a large family.[30]

4) Many people *believe* that couples today *do not need children* as did couples in previous generations. Fulfillment for both members of the family can be found outside the home. Moreover, children are not usually needed to support a family business or to care for their parents when they reach old age.[31]

5) *Couples whose relationship is weak* often see children as one more strain which might break the marriage.[32] It is not that children in themselves pose a threat, but rather that the demands they make on the couple's life style are seen as dangerous to the relationship. For children pose a problem for the wife's working, for making a budget stretch, for facing periods of unemployment, and for pursuing activities outside the home.

6) Wives who work after marriage and limit their family size do so *more to meet financial pressures than to further their careers.*[33]

It would be a mistake to presume that sociological studies can actually show that artificial contraception causes contemporary attitudes and life-styles, nor is the reverse situation proven true. *The most we can say is that these studies would be consistent with the conclusion of many that such is indeed the case.*

Has Contraception Promoted Sexual Permissiveness and Abortion?

Many people make what seems to them a solid judgement of common sense: the availability and acceptability of artificial contraception has caused an increase of premarital relations, cohabitation, and abortion. *Such a judgement may very well be correct, but once again, sociological research is far from adequate to settle this point.*

According to one study, a girl's decision about engaging in premarital sexual actions seems to be most dependent on her having a satisfactory relationship with her mother. Where such a relationship is present the girl is very likely to model herself after her mother, no matter what kind of model the other presents.[34] The availability and social acceptance of artificial contraception would seem to be only a *secondary* factor in such a girl's thinking.

Another study shows that many teenagers who are sexually active are either totally ignorant of contraceptive techniques or else use them inconsistently and carelessly.[35] If such is the case, then it would seem that the decision to be sexually active *precedes* any serious consideration of contraceptive use.

Studies show that couples who live together "without benefit of clergy" usually want few, if any, children in their lives; and so they will resort to artificial contraception. Their aversion to having children, however, *probably existed prior to* their seeking out modern contraceptive techniques.[36] The greater incidence of cohabitation today does indeed parallel the rise of contraceptive usage, but once again, we cannot assume that contraceptives are the *cause*, or at least the *total* cause of such cohabitation. Instead, the decision to live together may itself be the first serious occasion for a couple's selecting some means of artificial contraception.

Has the availability and social acceptance of artificial contraception contributed to the rise in abortions? Studies seem to indicate that the answer is not a simple yes or no. The rise in abortion may be traceable rather to the *failure* of contraceptive practice because of either their inherent limitations, or the carelessness of their users. There is evidence, for instance, of considerable haphazardness in the use of contraceptives, especially among teenagers. Women college students were initially quite aggressive and accurate in their use of contraception in the late 60's. Studies in 1973, however, and again in 1978 indicate that many college students were becoming more and more careless about effective contraception.[37] One might conclude that *this increasingly nonchalant attitude may indeed have been caused by the ever easier access to abortion as "back-up contraception."* One might also conclude, perhaps quite accurately, that an *irresponsible* element *in the contraceptive mentality* easily passes over *into the area of abortion.* Sociological studies, however, would not by themselves be capable of substantiating conclusions of this type.

Conclusion

There remain many questions about the effects artificial contraception has had and is likely to have on the physical health and the personal attitudes of the American public. Those who oppose artificial contraception and those who favor it would be wise to seek more and more insight into what artificial contraception is in fact bringing about in the lives of men and women today.

Discussion Questions

1. Are sociological studies of the relationship between artificial contraception and a deterioration of morals adequate at this point?
2. Sociological studies show that two or more different things are going on in society, e.g., people are both smoking more and having more automobile accidents. Can such studies *prove* that one thing is *caused* by another? or only that they happen in the same period?
3. How many means of artificial "contraception" often may not prevent conception at all, but cause an abortion?
4. Under what circumstances is "the pill" user 128 times more likely to have a heart attack than a non-user?
5. Do most working wives put off having children because they want a career?

Notes

1. U.S. Food and Drug Administration, detailed patient labeling leaflet on contraception, April 1978.

2. *Ibid.*

3. L. Darveen, "Injectible contraception in rural Bangladesh," *Lancet,* 5 November 1977, pp. 846–848.

4. R. P. Marwool and V. Beral, "Disappearance of spermatozoa in human ejaculate after vasectomy," *British Medical Journal, 1979, 1:87, 13.*

5. "Intrauterine Devices—Physicology" in *The Merck Manual,* 13th edition (Rahaway, Merck, 1977), pp. 927; and "Intrauterine Device Usage and Fetal Loss," *Obstetrics and Gynecology,* December 1981, Vol. 36, no. 6.

6. Evelyn Billings and Anna Westmore, *The Billings Method* (Victoria, Australia, O'Donovan, 1980, p. 159.

7. Darveen, *op. cit.*

8. Billings, *op. cit.,* p. 179.

9. L. Dennerstein *et al., Gynecology, Sex, and Psyche* (Melbourne, University, 1978), p. 172.

10. A. Rosenfeld, "Oral and Uterine Contraception: A 1978 risk assessment," *American Journal of Obstetrics and Gynecology,* 132:92, 1978.

11. U.S. Center for Disease Control, "Increased risk of hepatocellular adenoma in women with long-term use of oral contraceptives," *Morbidity and Mortality Weekly,* Rep. 26:293, 1977.

12. *World Health,* World Health Organization on Research in Family Planning, August–September, 1978, p. 29.

13. Billings, *op. cit.,* p. 174.

14. Rosenfeld, *op. cit.,* p. 100.

15. Howard W. Ory, "A Review of the Association between Intrauterine Devices and Acute Pelvic Inflammatory Disease." *The Journal of Reproductive Medicine.* April 4, 1978,

pp. 200–204; Ronald T. Burkman and the Women's Health Study, "Association Between Intrauterine Device and Pelvic Inflammatory Disease," in *Journal of the American College of Obstetricians and Gynecologists*, 1981, Vol. 57, n. 3, pp. 269–276.

16. Rosenfeld, *op.cit.*, p. 101.

17. Billings, *op. cit.*, p. 178.

18. U.S. Food and Drug Administration leaflet, *Op.cit.*

19. Dennerstein *et al.*, *op. cit.*, p. 172.

20. P. Jouannet, "Evolution of the Properties of Semen Immediately Following Vasectomy," *Journal of Reproductive Fertility*, April 1978.

21. Dr. Malcolm Carruthers, Hood, Clinical Laboratory Service, Mandsley Hospital and Institute of Psychiatry, London, in *Sun* newspaper, Melbourne, 1 May 1979.

22. R. P. Shearman, "Recent Advances in Contraception Technology" in *Medical Journal of Australia*, 2: 767–772, 1971; See also references above: Billings, p. 160–161; Shearman, p. 767–772; Darveen, p. 846–848; Dennerstein, p. 168.

23. J. R. Wilkie, "The Trend Toward Delayed Parenthood." *Journal of Marriage and the Family*, 1981, Vol. 43, pp. 583–591; "Digest" in International Family Planning Periodical.

24. B. Mindick and S. Oskamp, "Longitudinal Productive Research: An Approach to Methodological Studies in Studying Contraception," *Journal of Population*, 1979, 2, pp. 259–276.

25. L. Bouvier and S. Rao, Social religious *Factors in Fertility Decline* (Cambridge, Ballinger, 1975).

26. M. Nag, "Marriage and Kinship in Relation to Human Sexuality," in M. Nag *Population and Social Organizations* (The Hague, Paris, 1975).

27. N. Ryder, "The Character of Modern Fertility," in W. Peterson (ed.) *Readings in Population* (N.Y., Macmillan, 1972).

28. Ryder, *op. cit.*, and Bouvier and Rao, *op. cit.*

29. H. Feldman, "A Comparison of Intentional Parents and Intentionally Childless Couples," *Journal of Marriage and the Family*, 1981, Vol. 43, pp. 593–600.

30. Ryder, *op. cit.*

31. L. W. Hoffman and J. D. Manis, "The Value of Children in the United States: A New Approach to the Study of Fertility," *Journal of Marriage and Family*, 1979, Vol. 41, pp. 583–596.

32. N. Glenn and S. McLenahan, "Children and Marital Happiness: A Further Specification of the Relationship," *Journal of Marriage and the Family*, 1982, Vol. 44, pp. 63–72.

33. Wilke, *op. cit.*

34. J. Inezu and G. Fox, "Maternal Influence on the Sexual Behavior of Teen-Age Daughters," *Journal of Family Issues*. 1980, Vol. 1, pp. 81–102; Cf. also Theodora Ooms, ed., *Teenage Pregnancy in a Family Context* (Philadelphia Temple, 1981), p. 68, for rise in teenage venereal disease since 1956.

35. M. Rogel, "Contraceptive Behavior in Adolescence: A Decision-Making Perspective," *Journal of Youth and Adolescence*. 1980, Vol. 9, pp. 491–506.

36. P. R. Newcomb, "Cohabitation in America," *Journal of Marriage and the Family*. 1979, Vol. 41, pp. 597–603.

37. M. Gerrard, "Sex, Guilt, and Contraceptive Use," *Journal of Personality and Social Psychology*. 1982, Vol. 42, pp. 153–158.

Preview of
Chapter Ten

● In the 1970's disagreement with the Church's opposition to contraception was so broad-based that many people thought the teaching had actually changed.

● Pope John Paul II and the Synod of 1980 on Family Life reaffirmed the teaching against contraception.

● The two steps needed to understand the teaching are:

1) The nature of the person as an incarnate spirit means that fertility belongs to the whole person, not just the body.
2) Hence to intervene in the conjugal act to eliminate fertility changes and undermines the true significance of the conjugal act—depersonalizing it significantly.

● Couples are challenged to act freely and responsibly in respecting their conjugal intercourse—this requires prayer and sacrifice, but without the cross one cannot reach the resurrection.

CHAPTER 10

The Morality of Contraception and Sterilization

The health hazards of newly developed contraceptive and sterilizing medications and technologies raise genuine moral concerns. But this chapter will explore the more basic question: *does the deliberate use of contraception or sterilization destroy the moral goodness of an act of conjugal intercourse?*

Even to consider such a possibility seems far-fetched to many people, particularly those who have adopted the secular sexual ethics described in Chapter 6. In fact, preventing the conception of an unwanted child may seem to be a kind of moral imperative, regardless of what means of prevention are used.

Thus many Catholic couples are puzzled by the traditional Catholic objection to contraception and sterilization. They have heard that the Church approves the use of natural family planning for responsible parenthood. If the goal of family limitation is acceptable, what real difference does it make which means are used, natural or artificial?

Although abortion is widely practiced in cases of contraceptive failure, many people who approve contraception as "conception control" *do oppose* abortion as "birth control," for abortion does violence to a newly developing human being. But contraception and sterilization are practiced to *prevent* the unwelcome conception of a new human embryo.

After birth control pills were introduced in the 1950s, Pope John XXIII appointed a Pontifical Study Commission on Family Population and Birth Problems described above in Chapter 5. Some theologians were contending that the use of such pills should be approved as an acceptable method of extending the natural periods of infertility that natural family planning uses.

In fact, the Majority Report of this commission recommended that the Pope change traditional Catholic teaching to permit at least some forms of contraception, although a Minority Report vigorously opposed this.

Humanae Vitae and Controversy

After two years of further study and reflection Pope Paul VI issued his famous encyclical, *Humanae Vitae* ("Of Human Life") on July 29, 1968. This document reaffirms the Church's opposition to contraception and sterilization but it does so in the context of the teaching on conjugal love by the recently concluded Second Vatican Council.

During the long delay since Pope John XXIII had appointed the Study Commission, and especially after news of the Commission's Majority Report appeared in the press, *a widespread expectation of a change in the Church's teaching had built up.* Many couples had assumed that the teaching was doubtful and no longer fully obligatory.

In the decade of the 1970s disagreement with the teaching of *Humanae Vitae* was so broad-based among both theologians and lay Catholics that some scholars felt the teaching had been, in fact, modified by a kind of popular consensus in the Church. But when Pope John Paul II succeeded Pope Paul VI in 1978 he included the traditional doctrine as an integral part of his moral teaching in his worldwide pastoral journeys.

In October, 1980, the World Synod of Bishops met under the presidency of Pope John Paul II to discuss the problems of the Christian family. *Despite serious consideration of the opposition to the traditional teaching on contraception,* the Bishops of the Synod unanimously reaffirmed the teaching of *Humanae Vitae*. Pope John Paul II incorporated the basic consensus of the Synod into his "Apostolic Exhortation on the Family" *(Familiaris Consortio)* on November 22, 1981.

In this exhortation, Pope John Paul II appealed to theologians "to commit themselves to the task of illustrating ever more clearly the biblical foundations, the ethical grounds and the personalistic reasons behind this doctrine (of *Humanae Vitae*)."[1] The editors of this book believe it responds in a modest way to this request of the Holy Father.

The Second Vatican Council teaching on marriage in 1965 was cited in Chapter 5 as pointing out that the moral aspect of any procedure to control the transmission of life does not depend solely on sincere intentions or on an evaluation of motives, but must be determined by objective standards. The Council Fathers described these standards as "based on the nature of the human person and his or her acts" in order to "preserve the full sense of mutual self-giving and human procreation in the context of true love."[2]

Two steps must be taken to summarize the Church's moral teaching on contraception and sterilization in the light of the Council's fundamental point of departure. They are based on the nature of the person, and on the nature of the conjugal act and contraceptive intervention.

1) The Nature of the Person

Pope Paul VI in *Humanae Vitae* insisted on an "integral vision" of the human person including both person's earthly vocation and his supernatural and eternal vocation.[3]

Pope John Paul II speaks of the person as an "incarnate spirit, this is, a soul which expresses itself in a body and a body informed by an immortal spirit" so that "Love includes the human body, and the body is made a sharer in spiritual love."[4]

He adds, as already described in Chapter 5, "Consequently, sexuality . . . is by no means something purely biological, but concerns the innermost being of the human person as such." Human fertility is sometimes considered a purely biological function since it resembles the reproductive function of animals. But Pope John Paul II notes that human fertility "is directed to the generation of a human being, and so by its nature it surpasses the purely biological order and involves a whole series of personal values."[5]

In the Christian understanding of the person, human love can reflect the divine love within the Blessed Trinity. Hence conjugal love with its power to beget a child reflects the Trinity in a unique way.

122

2) The Nature of the Conjugal Act and Contraceptive Intervention

This second step builds upon human experience. Couples in love discover *two inherent meanings* in their conjugal act: The procreative and unitive. When they come together spontaneously for the marital act they simultaneously enter a uniquely unifying embrace and open themselves to the inherent capacity of their embrace for procreation. Their act is a *natural sacrament—a sign with two inherent meanings provided by God through nature.*

The key issue here concerns the morality of removing the procreative meaning from the marital embrace. Should couples not have the moral freedom to choose to render their embrace non-procreative as long as they respect its unitive meaning? Some Catholic ethicists in the birth control controversy argued that marriage *as a total covenant* should have a procreative meaning, but individual conjugal acts could be rendered non-procreative and performed simply as acts of unifying love.

The response to this proposal rests on the first step, the nature of the person. If the conjugal act reflects the body/spirit unity of the person, an intervention to eliminate its procreative potential affects both the persons who embrace and the personal self-giving they are performing. *They have not simply removed a biological component of their act.* They have changed the *personal nature* of their conjugal act. Or, to use a popular term, they have partially *depersonalized* their conjugal intercourse.

Chapter 5 described the integrist personalism used by recent Popes in making this judgment. Pope John Paul II reiterated Pope Paul VI's teaching on the inseparability of the two meanings of the conjugal act. He used language just as dramatic as the language of *depersonalization.* He spoke of couples who use contraception to separate the two meanings (unitive and procreative) that God has inscribed in their being and in the dynamism of their sexual communion. "They *degrade* human sexuality," he wrote, "and with it themselves and their married partner by altering its value of 'total' self-giving."[6]

Freedom and Nature

The two steps just presented as summarizing the Church's moral teaching on contraception and sterilization have not convinced everyone in the Church. *Perhaps the most common difficulty lies in the fact that most conjugal acts are infertile and do not actually have a procreative capacity, although they have a procreative significance.* Contraception seems only to extend natural infertility. Can that be "degrading" or "depersonalizing?"

At this point the crucial factor of human free decision enters. Consider this analogy: Some defective fetuses abort spontaneously; should not physicians be free to abort other defective fetuses? The answer is a firm "no" in the Judeo-Christian tradition. The point of the analogy is not to compare contraception and abortion which are morally different, but to compare the moral objections to choosing interventions which seem to extend what naturally occurs. Although nature provides infertile periods, the free decision to suppress fertility remains objectionable.

In the order of nature couples are bonded together by frequent acts of conjugal intercourse, although many such acts are infertile. Yet even the actual infertile acts *signify* a conjugal love which is both unitive and procreative in its full and complete realization. By these acts the couple *signify* both their love and the potentially procreative outcome of their love.

In practicing natural family planning for the good of their family, couples preserve the full *significance* of their conjugal acts. They choose freely to perform them. Even if they choose an infertile time in their fertility cycle, *they also choose to avoid any intervention to suppress fertility and deny the procreative significance of their conjugal act.* Their act is a true and authentic act of sexual love.

On the other hand, if they choose to intervene to eliminate the procreative significance of their act, it is no longer an authentic expression of true marital love. In fact, while the act might be motivated by love, one can say that the elimination of procreativity eliminates the full heterosexual meaning of human sexuality itself. In this sense, the contracepted act is not an act of true *sexual* love any more than a homosexual act is.

Thus Pope John Paul II wrote that the difference between contraception and natural family planning involves "two irreconcilable concepts of the human person and of human sexuality." He pointed out that in natural family planning "sexuality is respected and promoted in its truly and fully human dimension and is never 'used' as an 'object' that, by breaking the personal unity of soul and body, strikes at God's creation itself at the level of the deepest interaction of nature and person."[7]

The Pope is opposing a freely chosen elimination of the procreative *significance* of conjugal intercourse even though nature herself does not continually provide an actual procreative *capacity* in every marital act. Only in the twentieth century has modern science developed an extensive panoply of scientific techniques for eliminating the procreative capacity of the conjugal act. This has precipitated the worldwide controversy in which not only proponents of secular sexual ethics but many representatives of the Judeo-Christian tradition have accepted contraception for family planning.

Chapter 6 noted the way ethical proportionalists would justify some instances of contraception as premoral or ontic evil rather than moral evil. This does not mean that all who challenge the traditional teaching on contraception adopt proportionalism. *In any case, much disagreement exists and will not disappear overnight.* One scholar predicts that eventually the traditional teaching will be generally affirmed but only after patient dialogue and education similar to that which moves people to reject racial discrimination or segregation.

This teaching has not been solemnly defined by the Catholic Church with the claim of infallible truth which accompanies such statements. Yet the formal reaffirmations of the teaching in *Humanae Vitae* and, more recently, in the World Synod of 1980 and in *Familiaris Consortio* of Pope John Paul II, are significant. This constant teaching of recent popes and bishops after so much discussion seems a strong sign that the principles on which this teaching rests are revealed by God and could be solemnly defined as infallibly true.[8]

Practical Difficulties

Chapter 8 offered an overview of natural family planning as enriching marriages. Yet this presumes motivation and instruction which go hand in hand. In the face of the worldwide confusion and controversy on this issue, couples will not always discover the motivation and attain the instruction. They will find their way along this difficult path in vastly different ways. Couples facing the challenge of family planning were encouraged by Pope John Paul II at the end of the 1980 World Synod to make step-by-step progress in strength of conviction and in moral growth. This step-by-step progress, which everyone needs in dealing with his or her character deficiencies of any and all kinds (not just sexual ones), the pope called "law of gradualness."[9]

The Pope distinguished this from, and rejected, the idea of "gradualness of the law." This notion supposes different degrees or forms of obligation in God's law for different individuals and situations. Thus, a couple cannot say rightly: "Gradually—perhaps in a year or two—this moral law against contraception will take effect and we may *then* have an obligation to have another child or to practice NFP. But *right now*, this year, that moral law has not yet taken effect for us, and we are at this time free morally to use contraception." The Pope clearly sees no compromise in the core teaching for the inseparability of the two meanings of conjugal intercourse.

The U.S. Bishops in their 1976 pastoral reflection on the moral life recognized that conflicts and pressures on married couples can lessen their moral culpability when they use contraception. They encouraged couples not to lose heart or turn away from the community of faith when caught in these conflicts. The bishops urged them to do three things: to seek appropriate and understanding pastoral counsel, to make use of God's help in constant prayer and recourse to the sacraments; and to investigate natural family planning honestly and with open minds.[10]

Persons of faith know that children are the gift of God, just as the very act of conjugal love is also a gift. Pope Paul VI repeatedly refers to it as a divine gift in the key paragraph (#13) of *Humanae Vitae* on contraception. *To call it a gift means it is unmerited and bestowed on the couple, not merely a product of human achievement.*

Spouses are encouraged to assent to conjugal love and its unique manifestation in conjugal intercourse, much as one accepts a precious gift. Couples in love do not choose their delight in each other, they only assent to it. Each reflects God a bit more openly and unreservedly in their delight with the other. Over a period of months and years conjugal trust and gratitude for delight bestowed and enjoyed can and does deepen.

Yet marital chastity demands spiritual energy to defend unselfish love, described earlier in Chapter 8 as *agapeic* love, from the perils of selfishness and aggressiveness. It is understandable that sacrifice cannot be removed from family life, but must in fact be wholeheartedly accepted if the love between husband and wife is to be deepened and become a source of intimate joy. In Christian life as a whole, without the cross one cannot reach the resurrection.[11]

The Future

If the difficult and challenging doctrine on the integrity of conjugal love outlined here captures the minds and hearts of married couples, *the strongest single influence other than the grace of the Spirit, will be the example of other happy and loving couples.* In the discussion on natural family planning in Chapter 8 it was evident that married couples themselves are the most effective proponents of this doctrine.

Since the attitudes of most married couples toward conjugal activity and family planning are formed well before their marriage, the task facing the Church and diocesan leaders in the Family Life movement includes special emphasis on adolescents. Young people are forming their convictions about sexual ethics in the United States in a culture heavily influenced by secular sexual ethics.

The deeply divisive controversy over contraception in the last decade created what one author called, "The silence since *Humanae Vitae*." This silence led to a muffled witness to the ideals of Catholic sexual ethics in much religious education.

On the other hand, the Gospel brings Good News. In the case of family planning it offers a message of hope based on the genuine humanism of authentic conjugal love. In the troubled world of the 80's, for those searching for meaning in life and love, no more exciting ideal for marriage can be imagined than that proposed in the Good News of the Bible: *"Husbands, love your wives as Christ loved the Church."* (Eph. 5:25)

Discussion Questions

1. Can you outline the attitude toward contraception in the Catholic Church from the Second Vatican Council until the present?
2. What are the two steps which summarize the Church's moral teaching on contraception?
3. If a conjugal act has no actual capacity to procreate a child how does it still have a procreative significance?
4. Can you find the passage in chapter 6 where ethical proportionalism is applied to contraception? Why does Church teaching reject that approach?
5. What is the difference between "gradualism of the law" which Pope John Paul II rejected, and the "law of gradualness" which he accepted?
6. Can you think of instances of the "silence since *Humanae Vitae?*" How has the silence been broken, in your own experience?

Notes

1. *The Apostolic Exhortation on the Family (Familiaris Consortio)*. November 22, 1981, Vatican Text, #31.

2. *The Church in the Modern World (Gaudium et Spes)*, in *Vatican Council II. The Conciliar and Post Conciliar Documents*, ed. by Austin Flannery, O.P. (Collegeville, MN: The Liturgical Press, 1975), #51.

3. *Of Human Life (Humanae Vitae)*. July 29, 1968 (Huntington, IN: Our Sunday Visitor Inc., 1968), #7.

4. *The Apostolic Exhortation on the Family.* #11.

5. *Ibid.* #11.

6. *Ibid.* #32.

7. *Ibid.* #32.

8. Cf. Ford, John C., and Grisez, Germain, "Contraception and the Infallibility of the Ordinary Magisterium," *Theological Studies* 39 (June, 1978), n. 2, 258–312.

9. John Paul II, Homily at the close of the Sixth Synod of Bishops (October 25, 1980), 8: AAS 72 (1980), 1083.

10. "To Live in Christ Jesus," November 11, 1976, (Washington, D.C., U.S. Catholic Conference), p. 18.

11. Cf. *The Apostolic Exhortation of the Family.* #34.

Preview of
Chapter Eleven

● Contemporary genetic knowledge helps couples understand the degree of risk they may face in exercising their procreative gift in marriage.

● No evidence indicates an increase in the frequency of genetic disorders in the general population.

● Chromosomal imbalances are sometimes inherited but much more often arise when a defective sperm or ovum is produced or affected in some way.

● Tay-Sachs disease appears in ¼ of the children of two carrier parents, while ¼ are fully normal and the other half of the children are carriers.

● X-linked genetic defects occur in ½ of the male children when a parent has defective genes on the X chromosome. Some parents have chosen to abort any male fetus, even though ½ are normal.

● Neural tube defects result from defective genes and other factors and affect about one in 500 pregnancies.

Current Medical Knowledge of Genetic Defects

Using Catholic teaching and contemporary personalism, the previous chapter presented strong reasons for not intervening contraceptively in the act of conjugal intercourse. This chapter will focus on the procreative power of conjugal intercourse in the light of contemporary genetic knowledge according to which both parents contribute equally to the genetic makeup of their child. The next chapter will survey the moral issues which genetic medicine raises.

The concept of responsible parenthood described by Pope Paul VI in paragraph 10 of his famous encyclical, *Humanae Vitae (Of Human Life)*, includes knowledge and respect of the procreative power as well as prudent decision-making about the size of one's family. Pope Paul VI recognized that couples might make a legitimate and morally acceptable decision to avoid a new birth, even for an indeterminate period of time.

Could the significant risk of a genetically handicapped child provide an acceptable reason to avoid a new birth?

The Pope John XXIII Medical-Moral Research and Education Center formed a Task Force in 1976 to begin an exploration of moral issues in genetics. In 1980 it published a comprehensive report entitled *Genetic Counseling, the Church, and the Law.*[1] This study recognized that a couple might reach a responsible decision that it would be wrong to have additional children because of serious genetic risk, but it did not approve of abortion, sterilization, or contraception as means of avoiding a new birth. Genetic concerns can thus become a pressing reason for the knowledge and practice of natural family planning. (See Chapter 8.)

The Frequency of Genetic Disorders

No evidence indicates an increase in the actual numbers of genetic disorders during recent years, despite the contrary impression sometimes conveyed by some urging the importance of genetic counseling. However, the *relative* frequency and the *relative* importance of genetic disorders have increased dramatically in the last few decades.[2]

At the beginning of the 20th century, U.S. infant mortality was 150 deaths out of every 1,000 live births. Only about 5 of these 150 deaths, or 3.3%, were thought to be related to genetic causes. Since then many factors, including the introduction of antibiotic therapy and improved infant nutrition have dramatically decreased infant mortality. Today there are about 15 deaths for every 1,000 live births, a 90% reduction. Yet 5 of those 15 deaths, now a notable 33%, are still related to genetic causes.

About one-third of all admissions to children's hospitals are currently for birth defects; that is, for genetic diseases or diseases with some degree of genetic component. Patients with genetic diseases enter hospitals at least 5 times as often as patients with nongenetic diseases, and stay longer. Hence the burden of genetic disorders relative to other kinds of human illness *has* certainly increased.

In the U.S. population at large about 12 million persons suffer some form of birth defect with a genetic origin, although this includes minor as well as major abnormalities.[3] About 4% of liveborn infants have some sort of congenital malformation. Physicians are learning that an increasing number of familiar diseases such as hypertension, arterial chronic heart disease, and mental illness (schizophrenia and manic-depressive disorders) have a degree of genetic predisposition in some cases. Blue Cross/Blue Shield data show that about 20% of total U.S. health care costs are related to genetic diseases.

Chromosome abnormalities play an important role in miscarriages. It has been variously estimated that 15–70% of human conceptions are miscarried before birth, although some occur so early that a woman is unaware she has conceived. Among these miscarriages about 60% are chromosomally abnormal, which means that 10–40% of all conceptions are chromosomally abnormal. Hence the one child in 200 who is born with a chromosomal abnormality represents only a fraction of the total number of abnormal conceptions.

Chromosomal Imbalances

These chromosomal abnormalities result from errors in packaging the genetic material in the human cells.[4] No single gene is defective; rather, large numbers of genes have become scrambled, lost, or misplaced due to the absence or misplacement of a piece of chromosome. An entire chromosome may be missing; there may be extra chromosomes; or pieces from one chromosome may have gotten attached to a chromosome of another pair.

These defects can arise from abnormalities in the way cells differentiate and grow; they can be inherited from parents who are carriers; or they may occur when a defective sperm or ovum is produced or subjected to some change. For example, an ovum sometimes seems to suffer partial decay owing to the advanced age of a woman. Down's syndrome (mongolism) is one of the most common examples of a defect thought to arise from chromosomal imbalance.

The Pope John Center publication, *Genetic Counseling, the Church, and the Law,* presents a case study of possible chromosomal abnormality because of a mother's advanced age.[5] Mrs. M. was a pregnant woman 42 years old. She had been married since age 25 with no prior children or pregnancies. At age 27 she had had an ovary removed because of a cyst. She was told then that it was very unlikely she would ever become pregnant. She and her husband had not used birth control methods since that time.

She was about 3½ months pregnant when she went to a genetic counselor. She was aware of the increased risk that an older mother suffers of having a child with a chromosome anamoly. There was no prior family history of such a problem, although a first cousin had had a child with spina bifida, a condition in which the spine is incompletely formed.

Mrs. M. was told by the counselor that, while the incidence of Down's syndrome in an infant is about one in 500 births in the general population, it increases to one in 290 births from mothers in the age 35 to 39 year bracket, and to one in 100 births of mothers in her age bracket, ages 40 to 45. She was also told that her cousin's having a child with spina bifida did not significantly increase the risk of her having an affected child. The counselor also told her that no one can guarantee a normal child, and the risk of some significant abnormality at birth is between one in 50 to 100 births of all parents.

Mrs. M. was also informed of the availability of amniocentesis to provide samples of her amniotic fluid for chromosome tests and for testing for an increased level of alpha-fetoprotein which would indicate an incompletely formed spine. She chose to have amniocentesis. She said she was uncertain what she would do if the results were abnormal, although she suspected she would choose to abort.

The test results were available within four weeks. It should be noted that she was, by that time, approaching the middle of her second trimester of pregnancy. *If she were to choose an abortion, the fetus would already be nearing viability in the light of current achievements in neonatal intensive care.* Happily, the results of the amniocentesis were normal, the child was delivered safely, and did well.

This case of Mrs. M. amply illustrates subjective and personal aspects of the decision to perform amniocentesis and the possible abortion decision. Mrs. M. had no previous pregnancies, was approaching menopause, and would probably have used birth control had she realized she would become pregnant. Yet these subjective aspects do not change the moral evil of prenatal abortion for genetic defect. (See Chapter 12.)

Prenatal diagnosis for chromosomal imbalance is being performed rather widely today and the proportion of elective abortions in the case of positive indications of defect is extremely high.[6] An example of another genetic defect for which a select population of parents are at risk is Tay-Sachs disease.

Tay-Sachs Disease

Tay-Sachs disease results from the deficiency of an enzyme involved in the body process of breaking down a complex lipid (fatty material in human cells). The disease results from a progressive storage of undigested lipid in many tissues, but particularly in the brain. The enzyme deficiency which causes Tay-Sachs is traced to a gene which is defective. If that defective gene is paired with a normal gene, the usual process of breaking down the fatty lipid will ordinarily occur. *Hence this defect is described as a recessive genetic defect because it is hidden when paired with a normal gene.*

Those persons who have a defective gene responsible for Tay-Sachs are carriers of the condition even though they are themselves normal. If

132

two carrier parents have a child there will be three possible genetic outcomes. The child may inherit the defective gene from both parents, and inevitably suffer the disease. This will occur, statistically, in ¼ of the offspring. The child may inherit a defective gene from one parent and a normal gene from the other. This will occur in ½ of the offspring, and they will be carriers like their parents. Finally, the child may inherit a normal gene from both parents and would have no trace of the disease. This will occur in ¼ of the offspring.

The frequency of Tay-Sachs is much higher in the descendants of Eastern European Jews (Askenazi) than in other populations. Between ¹⁄₂₅ and ¹⁄₃₀ of this population are carriers of this gene. In intermarriages of this population the marriage of two carriers will occur about once in every 900 marriages. One-fourth of their offspring, or one in 3600 children of these marriages, will suffer Tay-Sachs.

In *Genetic Counseling, the Church, and the Law* the case of Mr. and Mrs. K. is presented. They are 56 and 58 years of age respectively.[7] Their first daughter, born when Mrs. K. was 22 years old, seemed completely normal until eight months of age when she failed to sit up and was considered retarded. Four months later physical and neurological tests suggested Tay-Sachs disease. The child regressed slowly but steadily and died at the age of three and a half, which is very commonly the life expectancy with this disease. During these years she developed gradual loss of motor function, weakness, blindness, inability to feed herself, frequent seizures similar to epilepsy, and, finally, she entered a comatose state.

The family suffered immensely as they watched the disease progress. *The shame they felt from carrying a defective gene that produced this disorder caused Mr. K to forbid his wife to divulge the diagnosis to anyone.* Years later their other daughter, born a year later than the one who had died, married and was expecting her first child. Mrs. K. divulged the secret to her daughter and son-in-law and they approached a genetic counselor.

Since Mr. and Mrs. K. had produced an affected child it was certain that they were *both* carriers. Their non-affected daughter had a ⅔ chance of being a carrier. Her husband, an Askenazi Jew like herself, had a ¹⁄₃₀ chance of being a carrier. That means the daughter had a ¹⁄₁₈₀ chance her unborn child would be a victim of the disease. Carrier testing is possible and so is prenatal diagnosis of the disease by amniocentesis.

In this case the daughter was identified as a carrier and her husband as a non-carrier. That meant that, on the average, half of their children would be carriers, but none would be affected because of the recessive character of the defect. The couple did not choose amniocentesis since they were assured that neither this child nor any subsequent children would be affected with Tay-Sachs.

The fact that therapeutic treatment for genetic disorders like Tay-Sachs or a chromosomal imbalance has not yet been discovered means that amniocentesis presently cannot lead to *prenatal* therapy in any but the rarest cases. It *can reassure* the large majority of women who are relieved to receive negative findings of the disorder. *But the very real temptation to abortion in the case of defect seems much stronger than in the case of healthy but unwanted fetuses.* One prestigious textbook in medical embryology even presents an option of two "medical approaches" in the face of genetic defect.[8] The options are postnatal repair, which is admittedly very limited in cases like Tay-Sachs, or early detection by prenatal diagnosis and abortion. The prolife philosophy so deeply rooted in the Judeo-Christian tradition and in Catholic teaching would describe these two options very simply as options of "caring or killing."

Dr. M. M. Kaback recently reported on his worldwide experience in Tay-Sachs testing.[9] About 250,000 carrier tests have been performed, about 210,000 in the U.S. Some 10,500 carriers were identified, with about 8,000 in the U.S. These figures were collected from 1969 to 1979, and out of this total screening experience, 210 couples were identified where both partners were carriers and were at risk of an affected child. Of these 210 couples, about 180 pregnancies were followed. *There were 32 positive diagnoses of the disease and 31 elective abortions performed.* From a group of 450 couples who already had had at least one Tay-Sachs child, *116 had affected fetuses and 111 were aborted.* Dr. Kaback insists, however, that no pressure is put on the parents to choose abortion. In fact, there are very strong groups among Orthodox Jews who are opposed to abortion under any circumstances.

X-Linked Genetic Defects

X-linked genetic defects have raised additional ethical concerns when an affected fetus is suspected. These genetic diseases result from abnormal genes on the X chromosome. Females have two X chromosomes, whereas males have a pairing of an X and a Y chromosome. Since females have two X's they are usually normal even if one of the X chromosomes is defective. But males have only one X chromosome and one Y chromosome and they will be affected if the one X chromosome they inherit is defective. A woman carrier of a defective X chromosome will have a 50% risk of producing an affected son and also a 50% risk of producing a carrier daughter.

The major X-linked disorders most frequently seen are muscular dystrophy (Duchenne's disease) and hemophilia, although some 109 X-linked disorders have now been recognized. Many of these conditions cannot be diagnosed prenatally. But prenatal sex determination can be made by amniocentesis. Hence some parents with a 50% risk of an affected son have chosen to abort any male fetus without knowing whether it is normal or affected, automatically destroying healthy as well as defective sons.

Neural Tube Defects

Another type of birth defect seems to result from complex conditions in which both defective genes and other factors are involved. The "neural tube defect" is a case in point.[10] Such defects are among the most common malformations of the central nervous system. They include anencephaly, which is the partial or complete absence of the cranial vault with either a complete absence of or only a rudimentary brain; encephalocele, which is the protrusion of the brain through the skull; and spina bifida, which is a defect in the closing of the neural arches in the lower spine.

Together, these malformations affect about one in 500 pregnancies in the general population. About half these instances are anencephaly which is fatal; the child is born dying if not stillborn. Encephalocele is generally fatal and infants who do survive are severely handicapped and mentally retarded. Spina bifida may not be fatal, depending on the size and location of the defect, whether the spine is open or closed, and what sort of complications occur during the neonatal period.

In 90% of the cases of neural tube defect there has not been a previously affected child. On the other hand, if there has been a previously affected child, the risk of recurrence is 2% to 3% in subsequent pregnancies. If a couple has had two children affected by spina bifida, the risk for a third child rises to about 5%. A person who has had spina bifida has about a 2% to a 3% risk of subsequently begetting a child with this condition. Normal brothers and sisters of an affected child have about a 1% risk of themselves having a child with a neural tube defect.[11]

Prenatal diagnosis of neural tube defects uses amniocentesis and measurement of alpha-fetoprotein levels. The false-negative rating is about 10% meaning that 10% of the instances will be missed, whereas the false-positive rating is quite low, about one in 1,000 cases. One clinic, combining alpha-fetoprotein and ultrasound studies, has attained a 100% accuracy in diagnosing neural tube defects over the past five years.[12]

135

Conclusion

Some small part of the information presented in this chapter will be inaccurate within a year or two simply because of the progress genetic medicine is making. Increased knowledge of genetic defects will eventually lead to better therapy and even to preventive treatment and the occurrence of these defects might actually diminish. *In the meantime, serious moral issues are raised by the use of abortion and contraception to prevent the birth of defective children.* The next chapter will explore those issues.

Discussion Questions

1. Is the incidence of genetic disorders increasing in the general population? Do many people think it is?
2. What is the frequency of birth of a Down's syndrome child in the general population? What is it among mothers aged 40 to 45? Do many people think it is more common among that age group than it actually is?
3. What is the difference between preventing birth defects and the births of defective children?
4. What causes Tay-Sachs disease? Is it fatal? Would a Tay-Sachs child be better off if a miscarriage had occurred?
5. Why would Mr. and Mrs. K. have been ashamed of having a defective child?
6. Why are X-linked disorders only passed on to sons and not to daughters? If abortion is performed, what proportion of healthy male fetuses are destroyed?
7. Can modern medicine provide genuinely therapeutic care for children with neural tube defects?

Notes

1. Atkinson, Gary M., and Moraczewski, Albert S., editors, *Genetic Counseling, the Church, and the Law*, (St. Louis, MO, The Pope John Center, 1980). This volume offers an invaluable supplement to Chapters 11 and 12 of this *Handbook*.
2. Cf. Moraczewski, Albert, Editor, *Genetic Medicine and Engineering, Ethical & Social Dimensions*, (St. Louis, MO, Catholic Health Association Publications, 1983), Chapter 1, in press.
3. Cf. Moraczewski, *op. cit.*, Chapter 2.
4. Cf. Atkinson and Moraczewski, *op cit.*, pp. 9–12.
5. *Ibid*, pp. 49–50.
6. Moraczewski, *op. cit.*, Chapter 4.
7. Atkinson and Moraczewski, *op. cit.*, pp. 32–34.

8. McCarthy, Donald, "The Either/Or of Genetic Defect" in *Ethics and Medics* (monthly newsletter of the Pope John Center), Mar. 1983, pp. 1–2.

9. Kaback, M. M., Nathan, T. J., and Greenwald, S., "Tay-Sachs Disease: Heterpzugpte Screening and Prenatal Diagnosis—U.S. Experience and World Perspective," *Tay-Sachs Disease: Screening and Prevention*, M. M. Kaback, ed. (New York: Alan R. Liss, 1977), pp. 13–36.

10. Cf. Monteleone, Patricia, and Moraczewski, Albert, "Medical and Ethical Aspects of the Prenatal Diagnosis of Genetic Disease," in *New Perspectives on Human Abortion* edited by Hilgers, Thomas W., Horan, Dennis J., and Wall, David, (Frederick, MD, University Publications of America, 1981), pp. 45–59.

11. Cf. Moraczewski, *op. cit.*, Chapter 2. Statistics given in Monteleone and Moraczewski, *op. cit.*, p. 52, indicate somewhat higher risks.

12. Cf. Moraczewski, *op. cit.*, Chapter 2.

Preview of
Chapter Twelve

● Genetic medicine is concerned with those diseases and disorders which are the result of inherited characteristics.

● Discussions of genetic defect cause prospective parents to review their attitude toward children as a gift, toward their notion of what it means to be human, and towards the role of suffering in human existence.

● Amniocentesis, a useful technique for gaining information about an unborn child, becomes immoral if used with the intention of aborting a defective child.

● Genetic counseling seeks to inform couples of their chances of conceiving a defective child.

● Treatment for genetic defects is extremely limited but prospects exist for future therapy even while the fetus is still in the womb.

CHAPTER 12

Moral Issues in Genetic Medicine

Introduction

While we are a long distance from made-to-order children, we have advanced considerably since Gregor Mendel first wrote the article in which he suggested that inherited traits were transmitted from one generation to the next as discrete units. These tiny packets of inherited characteristics are called genes. It was only after World War II that we began to recognize that these genes could be described biochemically in terms of the macromolecule, deoxyribonucleic acid (DNA). We have also broken "the genetic code," and now understand the chemical makeup of the genes themselves.

The genetic code determines the synthesis of many thousands of different proteins, a large proportion of which are enzymes. These in turn control the synthesis of hundreds of different substances which constitute the human body in structure and function.

Genetic medicine is concerned with those diseases and disorders which are the result of inherited characteristics. Diseases and disorders can be transmitted genetically in the same ways that other inherited characteristics are passed on. Genetic medicine deals with such anomalies, their causes and cures.

General Issues

There are three considerations which ought briefly to be reviewed because they set the foundation for the specific ethical issues which arise in genetic medicine; these are

1) The basic mind-set of a couple with regards to children
2) The Christian concept of the human
3) The attitude an individual has with regard to suffering, pain and disease.

Children—A Right or a Gift?

Married couples can view having children *as their right or as a privilege and gift from God.* In Catholic theology, as reflected in the Code of Canon Law, marriage confers a right to those *actions* which of themselves are designed for generation of children. Nowhere is it stated that couples have a right to the child itself. Indeed, Pope Pius XII explicitly denied that this is a right following upon marriage.[1] We do have a right, for example, to food in order to live; we have a right to education, to worship, to marriage in order to live as human beings. In contrast, we do not have a comparable right to a child because this would be saying, we have a right to own a person. To say that we have such a right would be tantamount to saying that a person rightfully can be a slave to another.

As a consequence of considering the child to be a right of the parents, there often follows the notion that the couple has a right to obtain a child by any means, including the use of artificial insemination, *in vitro* fertilization and surrogate parenting. (A more detailed discussion of these procedures will be found in Chapter 16.) Another false conclusion from that premise is that parents have a right to a healthy child. That conclusion leads to the further expectation that the child will be born perfect (without blemish of mind and body) by whatever standards are current. One consequence of such an attitude is that a child who is born less than perfect or who has a defect or disorder is likely to be rejected psychologically or even aborted.

140

In contrast, the Old Testament clearly upholds the principle that children are a gift of God. To have children was a blessing; not to have them, a curse. With her first child, Cain, Eve exclaimed, "I have produced a man with the help of the Lord." (Gn. 4:1) After Abel was slain by Cain, Eve's next child was Seth, which led her to say "God has granted me more offspring in place of Abel." (Gen. 4:25) Hannah, who was childless for many years, prayed to the Lord for a male child. Her request was granted and she returned to the temple with her son, Samuel, and told the priest, Eli, that "I prayed for this child and the Lord granted my request." (I Sam. 1:27) It was a request, not a demand that a right be fulfilled. These and numerous other references in the Old Testament all indicate that children were a gift of God, a blessing, not a right which a married couple could point to. The New Testament says nothing to change this Old Testament teaching.

What It Means To Be Human

Ethical considerations in genetic medicine are bound up with the meaning of what it is to be human. Clearly those who see human beings as creatures of God will interpret practical life situations differently from those who view humans as the sole judge of their own actions.

While the entire universe and its component parts are creatures of God, humans—by divine gift—hold a privileged position in the visible world.

What is man that you should be mindful of him,
or the son of man that you should care for him?

You have made him little less than the angels,
and crowned him with glory and honor.

You have given him rule over the works of your hands,
putting all things under his feet.
(Ps. 8:5–7)

Basic to the gift of human dignity, and subsequently perfected in Jesus Christ, is the human capability of entering into intimate friendship with God. Human beings are known by God—as all creatures are—and also able to know God, not only as He is reflected in creation (see Dn. 3:52–58) but also more directly in His Son, Jesus Christ. The Lord Jesus told the Pharisees, "If you knew me, you would know my Father

141

too." (Jn. 8:19) He also told Philip, "Whoever has seen me has seen the Father. How can you say, 'Show us the father'?" (Jn. 14:9) Ultimately, the Blessed in heaven see God face to face. (I Cor. 13:12)

Furthermore, the uniqueness of the human person does not begin when the individual is consciously aware of God. Rather that uniqueness starts in the womb.

> The word of the LORD came to me thus:
> Before I formed you in the womb I knew you,
> before you were born I dedicated you,
> a prophet to the nations I appointed you. (Jer. 1:4–5)

> Truly you have formed my inmost being;
> you knit me in my mother's womb.
> I give you thanks that I am fearfully, wonderfully made;
> wonderful are your works.
> My soul also you knew full well;
> nor was my frame unknown to you
> When I was made in secret,
> when I was fashioned in the depths of the earth.
> Your eyes have seen my actions;
> in your book they are all written;·
> my days were limited before one of them existed.
> (Ps. 139:13–16).

Official teachings of the Church have reinforced this basic Biblical view and insisted that human life from conception onwards is sacred.

The Christian view of human persons is that they are created and redeemed by God, that they have a responsible stewardship over the world, themselves and the children given to them, and that they have a personal and eternal destiny which transcends the present—a destiny in which the injustices and shortcomings of this world are rectified.

The Role of Suffering and Pain

The third general consideration is the role of suffering and pain in the life of a Christian. For many people, especially those not sharing rightly in the Christian outlook, suffering and pain are viewed as something totally wasteful and utterly to be rejected. In contrast, the Christian, reflecting on the cross of Christ, recognizes that suffering can be a response to the invitation of the Savior to take up one's cross daily. (Mt. 16:24)

The suffering encountered in the area of genetics is, in part, that experienced by the individual afflicted with a hereditary disorder. Whether it be physical pain or discomfort, or mental disability, or emotional illness such as some types of schizophrenia or manic-depression, the suffering is real and often permanent.

Suffering is also experienced by the parents who sometimes blame themselves for the condition of the child. Jesus anticipated this concern when he denied that the parents' sins are responsible for a person being born blind. Rather, he counseled that it be viewed in a larger setting of God's providential love:

> As he walked along, he saw a man who had been blind from birth. His disciples asked him, "Rabbi, was it his sin or that of his parents that caused him to be born blind?"
> "Neither," answered Jesus:
> "It was no sin, either of this man or of his parents.
> Rather, it was to let God's works show forth in him. (Jn. 9:1–3)

A Christian, then, will not respond to a genetic disease as an unmitigated calamity but will strive to evaluate it against the background of Jesus's life and his teachings regarding suffering.[2]

By no means should this teaching be taken as recommending a passive attitude towards illness, pain or suffering. Rather, we ought to do what we can and may to cure the illness, correct the dysfunction and relieve the pain.

Specific Issues

The following discussion of genetic medicine will consider three aspects of the field: *Diagnosis, counseling, and treatment.* Although these topics overlap to some extent, the division is useful for the orderly presentation of the moral issues most relevant to medical genetics.

Genetic Diagnosis

By the term *genetic diagnosis* we mean the procedures which are used in order to determine whether the unborn child has a particular genetic disease or whether the parent is a carrier of a specific disorder. This includes the estimation of the possibility that a particular individual or couple might have a child with a specific genetic disorder. Gener-

143

ally, there is no major moral problem with merely taking a person's history, or in sampling the blood for specific characteristics that would reveal some genetic disorder. The major concern in this area pertains to diagnostic procedures which are used on a pregnant woman in order to determine the condition of the unborn child. The three procedures which are currently most likely to raise ethical issues are those of amniocentesis, chorionic villi testing and fetoscopy.

Amniocentesis is the diagnostic technique by which a needle is inserted into the amniotic sac of the pregnant woman, sometime between the 14th and 16th week of pregnancy, in order to obtain a sample of amniotic fluid. This fluid contains, among other substances, cells which have been sloughed off the body surfaces of the unborn child. It is possible to detect a large variety of genetic disorders by a study of the chromosomes of these cells and of certain of their biochemical components.

Chorionic villi testing consists of surgically clipping off one of the hair-like villi which protrude from the outer surface of the amniotic sac. Laboratory examination of these villi can reveal genetic defects of the fetal child.

The chief moral problem surrounding amniocentesis and chorionic villi testing arises from two facts: 1) These procedures often lead to an elective abortion after a *positive* diagnosis, 2) The procedures themselves may induce a miscarriage or can injure the unborn child in a variety of ways. Catholic teaching has repeatedly stated that abortion is totally unacceptable.[3–4] *Therefore, if amniocentesis is done with the intention of aborting the child should the results indicate a genetic defect, it would be immoral.* If, however, there is no intention of opting for abortion, another problem emerges: The unborn child is subjected to at least some risk of injury by the procedure itself. Do these possible injuries override the expected benefit of the procedure? Considerable controversy exists as to the degree of risk. However, if the information obtained does not lead to any true benefit for the child, such as the institution of treatment procedures in utero, it would be difficult to justify any risk. The moral principle which is operative here is that the child may not be subjected to risks unless they are balanced by realistically estimated benefits, not for someone else, but for the infant.

The third diagnostic procedure to be considered here is that of *fetoscopy.* This is a technique which involves the insertion of a small diameter tube through the abdominal wall of the pregnant woman and into the amniotic cavity. Ultrasound scanning is used to guide the insertion and to avoid puncturing the fetus. By means of fiberoptics the child within the uterus can be directly observed. This permits the finding of a fetal blood vessel and obtaining a sample of blood for diagnostic purposes, or the performing of a biopsy. This procedure, to date, presents more risks than amniocentesis and many physicians hesitate doing it without a serious reason. They fear that the potential damage to the child is greater than the anticipated benefits. Such damage includes a significant increase in the rate of miscarriages as a result of the procedure itself. Consequently, *it seems difficult to justify morally the procedure of fetoscopy except in rather exceptional circumstances.*

Genetic Counseling

Before Pregnancy

If couples or individuals seek genetic counseling before the woman becomes pregnant, they are most often concerned about their chances of begetting a genetically defective child. Since these are frequently high risk situations, it is quite likely that they will be counseled to seek contraceptive sterilization. The teaching of the Church has been quite clear that no medical reasons can justify direct contraceptive sterilization. (See Chapter 10) However, there are realistic and effective alternatives today, namely, natural family planning methods (NFP). (See Chapter 8) *These methods have greatly improved in the last few years and offer morally acceptable and effective procedures which at the same time do not present any medical risks.*

Another procedure proposed as a means of avoiding the procreation of a child with a specific genetic disorder is that of artificial insemination with donor semen (AID). When it is determined that the husband is the carrier of the genetic disease, and yet the couple wish a child who is biologically related to the wife, this is the procedure often suggested. Pope Pius XII has been very vigorous in condemning AID and pointing out that it is immoral and " . . . to be summarily rejected."[5]

Some have proposed *in vitro* fertilization (IVF) as a means of dealing with the problem when the wife is the person with the genetic disorder. In those cases the egg is obtained from another woman and the husband provides the semen for fertilization. The resulting embryo is then implanted in his wife. This, too, is morally objectionable. The objection rests not merely on the fact that the semen ordinarily is obtained by masturbation. More fundamentally it rests on the fact that the egg is not his wife's and the procreating of new life has involved the intrusion of a necessary element (the egg) from outside the marriage covenant.

A third procedure which is basically a modification of AID and IVF is surrogate parenting. Here, a donated egg or donated sperm, or both, are brought together and the resulting embryo implanted in a woman who is not the wife. At term, this woman turns over the child to the couple desiring the infant. *In addition to the objections already raised with procedures that replace the marital act in begetting children, other problems also surface.* The procedure is bound to have a great effect upon the child. The surrogate mother may have difficulty in relinquishing the child. There is also the issue of what to do if the child is genetically defective. Will both the surrogate mother and the couple "ordering" the child reject it?

After Pregnancy

A different type of moral problem arises if the woman is already pregnant and the child is known to have a genetic disorder. *Abortion is often recommended in such cases. Clearly this is not morally acceptable.* This process is initiated by proposing amniocentesis as a diagnostic procedure. For reasons discussed above, the use of amniocentesis has severe limitations. (There are some situations where amniocentesis may be warranted. The technique, for example, may be used to determine the fetal maturity or the condition of the fetus in the presence of Rh incompatibility. The information would be of direct benefit to the unborn child, in that it would help determine the immediate steps possible, including early delivery, if the maturity of the child would warrant it.)

Another problem arising from this diagnostic procedure is that at times information may be withheld from the person. An individual has a right to know his or her condition, especially when they have approached a specialist to get that information. There may be times, however, when such information may be of no use and may actually bring about a problem.

Still another issue is that confidentiality may be violated. Generally, the physician-patient bond of confidentiality is considered inviolate. There are conditions when the individual may discover before marriage, for example, that he has, or is a carrier of, a serious genetic disease. The individual may decide to withhold such information from the intended spouse to prevent the marriage's being called off.

Counselors who have knowledge of this genetic disease are caught in a dilemma. They know that a third party can be injured by not having the knowledge. Because of the great importance of maintaining confidentiality, it is generally recognized that counselors usually are not obliged to inform the third party of the situation. However, the counselor is under obligation to do all he or she can to induce the person in question to share that information with others who would benefit thereby and who might be harmed by not having it.

146

Treatment for Genetic Defects

Unfortunately, there is not much that can be done about correcting genetic defects at the present time. Some steps can be taken to correct the symptoms, as in phenylketonuria (PKU) where, by strict dietary control at birth, the degree of mental retardation can be greatly reduced. At times surgical corrections of malformations can help to reduce some of the symptoms of a variety of genetic diseases. More recently, it has become possible to carry on surgical corrections *in utero.* Considerable experimentation has been done with monkeys in the area of hydrocephalus by introducing a stainless steel valve into the skull of an unborn monkey with hydrocephalus. This valve allowed fluid to drain from the cranial cavity and thus reduced the pressure on the brain.

Other experiments with fetal monkeys were directed to intrauterine repair of open neural tube defects (in humans also called spina bifida) by using a paste made of powdered bone to close the opening. Such experiments hold out the promise that some of these genetic disorders can be corrected earlier and more thoroughly in the future.

Clearly, the more desirable situation would be to prevent the disease or to correct the genetic defect at the level of the gene. While some progress has been made in this direction, human application at this time is extremely limited. According to our present knowledge and capabilities, direct manipulation of the defective gene would have to be done on the very young embryo. The only way in which this can presently be done would involve modifying the embryo *in vitro* before implantation in the uterus. It does not seem possible to reconcile the *in vitro* reproduction of human beings with the Church's oft repeated magisterial teaching on the nature and conditions of human procreation. (For fuller discussion of this point see Chapter 17.)

Moral analysis of intra-uterine treatment procedures would have to consider the relative risks. Reasonably foreseen risks would have to be weighed against expected benefits. At this moment, it is still relatively rare that treatment can be done *in utero.* However, modern technology in this area is developing quite rapidly. With carefully planned and executed animal experiments, sufficient knowledge and technical skill can be gained to make the introduction of such new techniques into human medicine morally acceptable.

Conclusion

Genetic medicine has come a long way in this century, especially in the last 25 years. As with all technology, however, medical progress is not without some moral problems. Pope John Paul II has repeatedly insisted that any technology which impacts on human beings is to be welcomed insofar as it truly benefits the individuals on whom it is used. At the same time, the technology and its effects must be weighed in the light of Christian moral principles so that human life is never exploited but is respected and perfected.

The suffering and disappointment of being childless or of having a severely handicapped child as a result of genetic disorder can be borne patiently with quiet Christian joy when experienced in faith as a part of God's loving providence. *To see in each person—whether unborn, mentally retarded, or otherwise handicapped—a redeemed child of God provides a powerful means of combating the secular humanistic ethic that would destroy or reject such individuals.* A solid foundation of faith permits the development and use of a genetic medicine that saves rather than destroys, that corrects rather than eliminates, that enhances rather than forsakes.

Discussion Questions

1. Why should we not say parents have a right to children? What do they have a right to?
2. What is the Christian view of a human person?
3. Did Jesus ever point to suffering and say it was *not* the result of sin? When?
4. When would it be immoral to have an amniocentesis performed?
5. What would be some situations where a couple might feel obligated not to have a child? (Refer back to the Tay-Sachs discussion of Chapter 11.)
6. Is abortion of a defective child any different, morally, than abortion of a healthy child?
7. Can you think of any situations where a genetic counselor would be tempted to reveal confidential information learned in a professional capacity?

Notes

1. Pius XII (1956) Address to the Second World Congress on Fertility and Sterility, May 20, 1956. English translation in *The Pope Speaks* (3):193–5, 1957.

2. See discussion on suffering in *Genetic Counseling, The Church and The Law*, Gary M. Atkinson & Albert S. Moraczewski, OP, Editors, (St. Louis: Pope John Center, 1980), pp. 80–85.

3. Sacred Congregation for the Doctrine of the Faith, English translation, *The Pope Speaks*, 19(3) 250–62, 1975.

4. Declaration on Abortion, Nov. 18, 1974, Washington, D.C.: U.S. Catholic Conference.

5. Piux XII, Address to the Fourth International Congress of Catholic Doctors, Sept. 29, 1949. English Translation in *The Human Body: Papal Teachings*, (Boston: Daughters of St. Paul, 1960), p. 118.

Preview of
Chapter Thirteen

● A person's male or female gender depends primarily on certain psychological aspects of their personality, whereas their male or female sex depends on anatomy and physiology.

● A child may be born with ambiguous anatomical sex; it becomes important to adopt a "sex of rearing" so the child's gender identity may properly develop. If surgical procedures assist the child in developing its own gender, they can be ethically recommended as corrective surgery.

● Transsexual persons are of one sex anatomically but perceive themselves to be of the opposite gender.

● To justify transsexual surgery in the light of Catholic teaching on the body/spirit unity, one would have to show that the anatomical sexual organs must be sacrificed as pathological in some sense or a threat to the health and well-being of the person. It seems very difficult to establish this.

CHAPTER 13

Therapy for Persons of Ambiguous Sexual Identity

Introduction

Occasionally a child is born who is not clearly a boy or girl when first seen at the time of delivery. Ordinarily, the nurse or physician is able to inform the new mother and the anxious father that they are now the proud parents of a baby boy or baby girl. However, sometimes it happens that this identification cannot be readily determined because the baby's sex organs are not clearly male or female. These organs are called *ambiguous genitalia* (AG). Individuals with this problem are persons with an ambiguous genital identity. Are they male or female, man or woman, both or neither?

Another type of confusion regarding genital identity is the situation *where individuals anatomically are clearly male or female, but feel, and indeed are convinced, that they are in the inner core of their being the opposite gender*

151

from that which their anatomy would signify. While having male genitalia, the individual perceives herself to be a woman or, having female genitalia, the person sees himself as really being a man. Such individuals are said to be transsexuals.

In all these situations there is some doubt about the relationship of gender and sex. *Gender* refers primarily to the psychological aspects of man and woman. *Sex* is a physiological and anatomical term and describes the individual as male or female.

Until very recently it was thought that sex and gender were tightly coupled: that if an individual had, for example, male anatomy, the individual was necessarily of human male gender—a man. Similarly, a person with female anatomy was necessarily of female gender—a woman. Down through the centuries it has always been known, however, that "errors" can take place during embryological sexual development. For example, what gender would a true hermaphrodite be? This individual has both male and female anatomy: breasts, functioning ovarian tissue, functioning testicular tissue, a phallus, a vagina and uterus. Is the person a male or female, a man or a woman? Another example is the sex reversal syndrome in which the individual's sex chromosomes are the opposite of what one would expect on the basis of their external and internal anatomy.

While the actual number of persons exhibiting disorders in sexual development is low, these cases are very important for a deeper understanding of what is meant by sex and gender and their interrelationship. *The abnormal contributes to a comprehensive understanding of the normal.*

There are a number of problems associated with these conditions: problems which are both medical and ethical. The problems are medical because the conditions require a correct diagnosis and a suitable treatment with drugs, surgery, and psychological counseling. They are ethical (and theological) because they raise profound questions regarding the nature of human sexuality and what chemical and surgical alterations may be done to the human body.

This chapter, then, will consider briefly the medical and ethical aspects of ambiguous genitalia and transsexualism *in order to provide some information about how a Christian faced with these kinds of problems may deal appropriately with the situation.*

Ambiguous Genitalia—Medical Aspects

The diagnosis of ambiguous genitalia is made when a penis and testes are not clearly discernible in a newborn child or when the clitoris is so enlarged as to suggest a penis. In either event the sex of the individual is not clearly shown in the external anatomy. A physician may find a case of ambiguous genitalia while examining an older person, even in the late teens or early 20s. Obviously, such ambiguity about genital identity raises a host of personal problems, especially if the individual is contemplating marriage.

Causes of Ambiguous Genitalia

The origin and genesis of ambiguous genitalia (AG) are not fully understood. Some of the probable causes of AG include environmental factors. These may be viruses which affect the development of the unborn child's gonads, or chemical substances administered to the mother during pregnancy. Other causes of the condition are abnormalities of the sex chromosomes or congenital defects.

What is not often appreciated is that the development of sexual organs is a rather complex process involving the interaction of a number of factors. For the first 6 to 8 weeks of development the embryo is neither male nor female; that is to say, the gonads are neither ovaries nor testes.

If the individual is a chromosomal male, then starting in the second month there results a series of biochemical steps leading to the conversion of the gonads into male genitalia.

If the embryo's chromosomes are those of a female, the gonads develop automatically into ovaries and no further action is necessary. *In other words, the formation of the female sexual anatomy is less complicated than that of the male sex.* More things can go wrong in producing the male genitalia.

Treatment

Experience has shown that the newborn who has ambiguous genitalia should not be sent home or given a name which subsequently may turn out to be inappropriate. Pediatricians who work in this field urge that the child be sent to an appropriate hospital where the team approach can be used to deal with this condition. The team should include a pediatric endocrinologist, a neurologist or general surgeon who is familiar with genital surgery, a radiologist, and a psychiatrist or psychologist. The purpose of this team is to offer the parents expert advice as to which sex would give the child the best chance to develop normally, with as little psychological stress as possible. In other words, they recommend what is called the "sex of rearing." This term refers to the sex in which the child will be raised. If the sex is to be female, then she is named appropriately and dressed suitably. The decision includes all aspects of her development, including the kind of gender model offered her for imitation. Once this is determined, it is important that all elements of the child's sex-role development further the decision made at birth.

If surgical correction is indicated, it should be done, if at all possible, before discharge from the hospital. Sometimes the surgery has to be done in several stages, so it should be scheduled before discharge and performed as quickly as possible.

Among the kinds of ambiguous genitalia, perhaps one of the most difficult to deal with is that of the individual with a micropenis. Micropenis, as the name suggests, is a condition in which the penis is so small that it cannot function as an organ of reproduction. In some cases the micropenis will respond to hormone therapy; however, if this does not take place and the penis remains very small, this should influence the decision regarding the sex of rearing. In this situation many experts hold that a female sex of rearing may best contribute to the psychological and social adjustments the child will have to make. Such a decision should be made early in life otherwise great difficulties for the individual are likely to arise.

Ambiguous Genitalia—Theological and Ethical Aspects

The fundamental question in the area of moral concerns is that of determining whether or not there exists an objective sex and gender. When the individual is conceived does he or she have a specific sex and gender? If so, how can this be decided?

Until very recently, it was thought that an individual who was equipped with a penis and testes was male; if these were absent the individual was necessarily a female. Then, because of situations where there was some ambiguity about the external genitalia, it was thought that chromosomes would be a better indicator of sex. A pair of X chromosomes would identify the female individual while an XY pair of chromosomes would constitute the male. That criterion held up only until it was discovered that there is a condition called the sex reversal syndrome where there are persons who are chromosomally male and anatomically female and vice versa. This made it most difficult to determine whether chromosomes were truly objective means of ascertaining sexual identity. *Perhaps the solution is to say that, in the vast majority of cases, XX chromosomes identify a female and XY the male. The ambiguous cases may point either to our limited knowledge or to a physiological ambiguity.*

Regarding a newborn child with ambiguous genitalia, the major ethical issue revolves around the sex of rearing. Studies have shown that gender identity is formed within the first 18–24 months of life. Consequently, it is crucial that the sex of rearing be determined as early as possible.

After assessing the total condition of the newborn child, the types of available corrective measures, and their likelihood of success, the medical team can provide the necessary technical and medical information and offer what they believe to be the best course of action to follow. But it is the parents that must decide whether or not to accept the recommended sex of rearing. The recommendations might include a surgical procedure so that there is no obvious anatomical sexual ambiguity when the child is growing up.

A more difficult decision arises when a male child has a micropenis which does not respond to testosterone therapy. If raised as a male, he will never be able to function sexually as a male. He could not assume the male position when urinating, nor could he achieve penetration if he attempted intercourse. These and associated limitations would ensure for him a life burdened by feelings of insecurity and awkwardness.

One medical approach which has been used is to remove the testes, and raise the child as a female. At puberty the child would be placed on estrogen therapy so as to bring about breast development. At the age of 18, the tissue of the external genitalia might be reconstructed so as to provide a vaginal pouch. In spite of the hormonal treatment and surgical reconstruction, the individual would not be able to bear children— not having ovaries or a uterus. Yet, the presumption made by those recommending this procedure is that the individual would function socially much better if accepted as a female than as a male.

Would this be an unjustifiable type of mutilation in the theological sense? If so, one could not ethically proceed along this path. There is a clear sexual ambiguity in some of these cases. Because of our limited knowledge regarding what precisely constitutes the individual's true sex, it is extremely difficult to determine whether the surgical and hormonal procedure described here is corrective in nature or an unjustified mutilation of the basic male identity of the person.

Since the question cannot be answered with certainty in at least some cases, the parents and physicians may proceed with whatever seems to offer the best chance for the person to find social acceptance. It must be stressed here that this is a provisional position based on the current stage of knowledge. Subsequent data may alter this analysis. It is also by no means clear that such a surgically altered person could enter a canonically valid marriage.

Transsexualism—Medical Aspects

A second major question may be stated as follows: Granted that an individual is *anatomically* clearly either a male or a female, does this necessarily mean that the person's *gender* identity is correspondingly that of a man or a woman? The condition of transsexualism raises the doubt. The fact that the doubt is raised does not necessarily mean the gender identity *truly is different* than the anatomical sexual identity.

The condition of transsexualism, however, raises a question about whether anatomical, physiological sex is tightly coupled with that of gender identity. Does male anatomy absolutely mean a masculine gender? Is it possible that, due to severe and unusual combinations of circumstances, an individual's physical sex does not correspond with his or her gender identity?

Diagnosis of Transsexualism

Those individuals are considered transsexual who anatomically are one sex but perceive themselves to be of the opposite gender. Such individuals do not doubt their anatomical identity. They are convinced it is the wrong one and therefore desire their anatomy to correspond with their perceived gender identity. The condition can become acutely painful, leading to severe disruption of their lives, and even suicidal tendencies.

Treatment of the Transsexual

Although public attention to this phenomenon dates to 1952 when press reports of Christine Jorgensen's surgical transformation took place in Denmark, there are apparently records of transsexual surgery in Germany dating back to 1919. The first United States program for transsexual surgery was opened at the Johns Hopkins Hospital in 1965. Since then it is estimated that some 6,000 persons in the United States have undergone transsexual surgery.[1]

Recommended treatment for the transsexual varies widely from doing nothing with the hope that eventually the experience of disharmony between gender and anatomy "will go away" to extensive surgical reconstruction on demand. *In between is the approach of psychotherapy which holds that eventually the patient is more likely to change his/her mind before changing his/her sexual anatomy.* There are also centers which have worked out programs for transsexuals involving several stages of treatment.

Because many, if not most, transsexuals are self-diagnosed, reputable treatment centers require a careful screening process and a trial period of living out the chosen sex role for one to two years before any surgical transformation is undertaken. The individual is required to dress and function socially in the role of the desired gender. Often this external change greatly reduces the inner tension which had caused so much mental anguish. On the basis of the original screening data and the results of the real-life test, the team then decides whether surgery is the recommended procedure. The individual, of course, has the final decision.

Male-to-female transsexuals receive estrogen during the real-life test. The primary effect of this hormone is to enlarge the breasts. There is some reduction in the size of the genitalia but no significant change in the voice. Female-to-male transsexuals receive the male hormone, testosterone. Menstrual periods end, the voice becomes lower and more hair grows on the face and other parts of the body.

Surgical reconstruction of the male-to-female transsexual is somewhat more satisfactory than the reverse. The testes are removed, the scrotum can be reshaped to form the labia, and after removal of the erectile tissue from the penis, its skin can be inverted to form a vagina-like pouch and placed in the normal female position.

For the female-to-male alteration, when desired, the vagina is closed and the labia are used to form a scrotum into which are placed prostheses of appropriate shape and size. Surgical construction of a penis-like appendage does not result in a convincing product, although a stiffening of the "penis" can be produced by suitable plastic prostheses.

In both instances—male-to-female, female-to-male—however, *the individual is not fertile as a member of the new gender role. Such individuals remain impotent in a canonical sense.*

Transsexualism—Theological and Ethical Aspects

The question of whether there is an objective measure for sex and gender was raised in the discussion of ambiguous genitalia. This consideration applies to transsexualism as well. *If* it were possible for a person objectively to be of one gender while being at the same time of the opposite anatomical and physiological sex, then in such a situation hormonal and surgical alterations *could* be seen as *corrective* rather than being an unjustifiable type of mutilation in the theological sense.

The problem, of course, is that at present there seems to be no convincing evidence that such a condition can exist. There are some indications that the basis for such evidence may exist in brain differences.

Animal and human data gathered in the last few years show that there are subtle but real differences in the brains of men and women. Whether these are related to gender as well as to sex is not clear.

Yet, because there are transsexuals—persons who sincerely and painfully believe that they are of a gender the opposite of that which their anatomy signifies—*the ethical implications of various therapies must be explored in the light of the Judeo-Christian tradition and Catholic teaching.*

Pope Pius XII clearly taught on more than one occasion that the principle of totality teaches that a functional part of the body must not be removed, destroyed or otherwise incapacitated unless necessary to preserve the health and well-being of the person as a whole. Hence, to change radically one's sexual anatomy might seem to be an unjustifiable type of mutilation, that is, one which would violate the principle of totality.

But, if the parts removed are seen as "pathological" in some sense, the surgical removal would not seem to violate this principle. Unfortunately, it seems very difficult to establish clear and convincing argumentation that the surgical removal of a transsexual's genital organs can be shown to be viewed in this light.

Both the transsexual person and the therapists may well be convinced that the surgery would be genuinely therapeutic. *Whether this justification can be sustained in the light of Catholic teaching about the person as a body/spirit unity remains dubious.* To sustain it, as mentioned above, one would need solid ground for judging the organs to be removed as pathological in some sense.

Even on practical grounds, a good number of experts believe that the sacrifice of bodily integrity in an effort to achieve a degree of mental stability is not justified. They say that the desire for a gender change is primarily psychological and that the proper treatment is psychotherapy not surgery.

"According to the data, a very high percentage of the persons asking for such surgery, if given adequate psychiatric help over one or two years, will no longer request it. As to those who do go through with surgery, there is some disagreement among the experts concerning its success . . . My personal judgment is that . . . these persons are yielding to an obsessive and illusory idea . . ."[2]

Conclusion

Clearly, in this matter of ambiguous genitalia and transsexualism there are as yet large areas of uncertainty. Because a child born with ambiguous genitalia will inevitably face problems in growing up, it is important that a decision be made as early and as competently as possible. To force a child to live out a gender life-style which will cause him severe embarrassment and social rejection would be ethically unacceptable. Every effort must be made to determine what the individual's true gender is in order to provide the basis for gender identity compatible with the manifest sexual anatomy.

The transsexual differs from the person with ambiguous genitalia not only because this individual is usually an adult but also because there is generally no confusion about the external genitalia. The confusion resides in the person perceiving a lack of harmony between his or her gender identity and sexual anatomy. Such a perception often results in an increasing mental anguish, sometimes leading to self-destruction. *At this time no clear and definitive moral decision in favor of transsexual surgery can be made because of the lack of convincing proof* that such disharmony does objectively exist and that transsexual surgery could be justified as corrective and therapeutic.

Discussion Questions

1. What is the difference between gender and sex?
2. How should specialists determine the "sex of rearing" of a child with ambiguous genitalia?
3. How could one justify surgery to remove a micropenis?
4. How would you describe the condition of a transsexual person?
5. What possible forms of treatment are available for a transsexual person?

Notes
1. See Paul A. Walker, "A Contemporary Perspective on Gender Dysphosia," in Moraczewski, Schwartz, and Monteleone, *Sex and Gender* (The Pope John Center, 1983), pp. 269–270.
2. Ashley, Benedict, "A Theological Overview on Recent Research on Sex and Gender", *Sex and Gender, cit.*, p. 42–43.

Preview of
Chapter Fourteen

● The homosexual orientation and behavior of persons covers a wide spectrum from temporary and minor inclinations to exclusive and deeply rooted patterns.

● Homosexuality is a complex phenomenon which cannot be completely correlated with effeminacy or a distant father-son relationship among males.

● No clear explanation of the cause(s) of the homosexual orientation has yet emerged, though the most popular theories trace it to early psychological development.

● Familial factors in early childhood are often suggested as influencing the homosexual orientation; if so, an ounce of prevention is worth a pound of cure.

● Treatment of homosexual persons to change an exclusively homosexual orientation offers little hope of success, but therapy can assist with developing self-esteem, controlling compulsive actions, and avoiding situations which foster homosexual activity.

160

CHAPTER 14

Homosexual Orientation and Behavior

A man would hardly come home to his wife and remark, *"I met a heterosexual in the drugstore when I was picking up a pack of cigarettes."* But he might well remark that he met a homosexual there. This indicates how readily a person can be categorized and identified if that person is different from the greater part of the population.

This chapter does not discuss homosexuals as if they were a different species from the rest of the population. It addresses homosexual orientation and behavior as found in various forms among people who are real and lovable persons just like all members of the human family.

Although sexuality is inherent in all aspects of life, human motivation and activity should not be explained entirely on the basis of sexuality. The labels, *heterosexual* and *homosexual*, are inadequate descriptions of human persons. This chapter will speak of *homosexual* persons, not simply *homosexuals*.

161

Homosexual behavior is not something new. It was recorded, for example, among the early Jews, Greeks, and Romans. Arlo Karlen has studied its history and notes that exclusively homosexual behavior was usually viewed negatively and was punished severely in many societies. If homosexual acts were accepted, it was *only* in special situations or at certain times of life.[1]

An indication that deep-rooted antipathy toward homosexual behavior can be found in modern society comes from a survey of 1000 physicians. Responding anonymously to a questionnaire, 75% of them acknowledged that knowing a male patient to have a homosexual orientation would adversely affect their medical relationship with the individual.[2]

This apparent bias among such a large sampling of physicians cannot be traced to any clearly and uniformly defined characteristics of homosexual persons. On the contrary, Dr. Alan Bell, a psychologist and professor of education at Indiana University, asserts flatly that there is no such thing as homosexuality.

He explains that the homosexual experience is so diverse and its originating factors so numerous that the term homosexual says nothing more about the person than that he or she can become erotically aroused by persons of the same sex or engages in sexual behavior with persons of the same sex.[3]

The word *homosexual* can refer to men or women. The first half of the word comes from the Greek word *homos,* meaning the same. Although *lesbian* is also a term used for female homosexual persons, *this discussion will use the term homosexual persons for both males and females unless otherwise stated.*

The term *homosexual* may describe a tendency or behavior covering a wide spectrum from the most temporary and minor inclinations of teenagers and young adults to permanent, exclusive, and deeply rooted patterns of homosexual preference in mature adults. Environmental factors such as found in boarding schools, prisons, and military assignments may influence the *degree* of conscious homosexual orientation a person experiences.

The Kinsey studies in 1948 created a numerical scale using the number 0 for persons of exclusively heterosexual orientation and ascending progressively to the number 6 for persons of exclusively homosexual orientation.[4] On this scale a person rated with the number 3 would be truly bisexual even though others might describe him or her as homosexual because of the evidence of strong homosexual tendencies. On this Kinsey Scale the extremes of exclusively heterosexual or homosexual behavior (numbers 0 and 6) are not the "normals" from a statistical viewpoint. Statistically, the normals would be numbers 1 and 5, which avoid the two extremes.

Studies of homosexual behavior based on small groups of subjects in prison populations or under clinical treatment give inadequate and incomplete information. *Studies of homosexuality which do not include heterosexual control groups are of little value.* Furthermore, the control group must match, as nearly as possible, the age, education, socioeconomic status, sex, and race of the group under study.

One helpful study of males with a homosexual orientation by Saghir and Robbins did use a control group of heterosexual persons and did reveal some significant data.[5] For instance, two-thirds of the males who were homosexual describe themselves as having been girl-like in their childhood, as opposed to only 3% of the males who were heterosexual. Of those who had been girl-like in childhood, 77% reported having had no male buddies, having played predominantly with girls, and having avoided boys' games. Those who were homosexual also seemed more concerned about their appearance than the control group.

A final significant point in this study showed that 84% of the homosexual males—as opposed to only 18% of the heterosexuals—reported that their fathers were indifferent to them or uninvolved with them in childhood. The fathers of the homosexual group were either physically or psychologically absent, rarely played with their sons, often dealt harshly with them, and sometimes called them nicknames that hurt their self-image and self-esteem. In these cases the mother seemed to replace the father as parent model and relations with the mother were close. The socioeconomic status of the parents seemed to make no significant difference.

Complexity of Homosexuality

However, one must be cautious about identifying homosexuality with any of these characteristics or circumstances. In the study above, for instance, one third of the male homosexual persons did not describe their outlook as girl-like in childhood. It should be noted, too, that almost ⅕th of the heterosexual persons did report a distant relationship with *their* fathers.

One cannot conclude, therefore, every male who seems effeminate or who was distant from his father in childhood has a homosexual orientation. *Some males in the study had a homosexual orientation despite close relationships with their fathers and a male-oriented outlook during childhood.*

Yet the correlation in the study between homosexual orientation and effeminacy and an inadequate father-son bond cannot be ignored. At the very least, it sends a clear signal to parents that boys need a good, strong relationship with both parents to develop an adult heterosexual orientation. It suggests also that encouraging young boys to begin early

163

in developing close relationships with other boys may strengthen a heterosexual orientation.

The fact that no definitive characteristics can be linked with *all* homosexual persons testifies to the complexity of both homosexuality and human personhood. Homosexuality is a complex phenomenon. Its manifestations in individual and social experience and behavior are quite complex, as are its biological and cultural aspects.[6] Another indication of complexity shows up in the variety of degrees of manifestation of homosexuality in the Kinsey study and others as well.

Researchers have distinguished between temporary and permanent homosexuality. Temporary homosexuality is shown in slight and occasionally acted-out tendencies toward homosexuality. The permanent orientation is deep-seated and sometimes even involves a clear aversion toward members of the opposite sex.

Some studies have also explored what they call "latent homosexuality." In the tradition of Freudian analysis, homosexual fantasies and impulses of males can be quite strong but suppressed, or "latent," in individuals with a bisexual constitution. These impulses can be attributed to an inherited feminine component in their personalities. Lionel Ovesey studies heterosexual males suffering dependency and power conflicts.[7] He found many "false" or "pseudo" homosexual motivations among them and used this model in psychotherapy with genuinely homosexual persons.

A priest-psychiatrist, Rev. Michael R. Peterson M.D., has pointed out that individuals may engage in heterosexual activity while the brain, as the seat of sexual fantasies and the source of erotic attraction, may show strong homosexual inclinations.[8] Dr. Peterson cites a case of a male professor of medicine who came to him at the age of 52 after 31 years of marriage and after raising six children. He had lost interest in marital intercourse but developed a sexual relationship with a male 19-year-old college student. In therapy it developed that the professor's fantasies for sexual arousal with his wife were almost exclusively involved with young boys and young men.

Homosexual Proportion of Population

Obviously, this discussion of the complexity of male homosexuality indicates the difficulty in estimating what proportion of the population are homosexual persons. The Kinsey study of 1948 reported that 37% of the total male population surveyed reported at least incidental homosexual activity to the point of orgasm at some time between adolescence and old age.

Furthermore, 25% reported more than incidental homosexual experience or reactions for at least three years between the ages of 16 and 55 years. About 18% reported at least as much homosexual as heterosexual behavior for at least three years, while 10% were more or less exclusively homosexual throughout their lives after the onset of adolescence. These data have since been reaffirmed in smaller studies.[9]

Estimates of the proportion of the total female population who are homosexual followed the same distribution pattern in the 1953 Kinsey study, but with a consistently lower proportion, averaging about one-half to two-thirds of the incidence for males. There seems to be much less overt homosexuality among women than among men, as well as less promiscuity and less homosexual prostitution.

A number of reasons have been proposed for the lower incidence of homosexuality among women. For instance, successful achievement of a feminine identity (not women's rights!) is considered easier, at least in western culture, than achieving a masculine identity. It is also easier, at least in western culture, than achieving a masculine identity. It is also easier in sexual relations for a woman to appear competent than for a man. Fewer studies have been done on female than male homosexuality, but one frequently occurring background factor was a strong anti-heterosexual pattern in the home, discouraging the daughters from associating with boys.

Sociological studies of homosexual persons have come a long way since Alfred Kinsey's pioneering surveys described here. Kinsey showed that the proportion of homosexual persons in the population is much higher than most people were willing to admit. His Kinsey Scale of sexual preference rating from 0 to 6 challenged the previous either-or-view of sexual orientation.

More recent studies indicate that a single scale like Kinsey's does not accurately portray sexual behavior and orientation. It has been suggested for example, that individuals could have a double rating. One might show their *homosexual* orientation, the other their *heterosexual* orientation. Another possible modification would rate a person on three different levels of sexual orientation: Sexual behavior, sexual fantasies, and affective preference. The last category would rate the person's choice for affection and intimacy. Conceivably, an individual could have homosexual behavior and fantasies but a heterosexual preference for affection and intimacy.

Another factor the Kinsey study did not uncover is the possibility of change in sexual orientation over time, since no follow-up was made with his sample population. It is unknown exactly how stable sexual orientation remains over time. It appears to be stable, but there are some indications that some individuals may experience a genuine, spontane-

165

ous change in sexual orientation over time. This is different from merely acknowledging long-suppressed homosexual feelings.

The meaning people find in sexual experience may also change over time, and this may affect behavior. This last possibility raises interesting prospects of the role a religious system of meaning and value might play in a homosexual person's directing sex preference as well as sexual behavior according to moral ideas.

Causes of the Homosexual Orientation

Despite the great number of studies of homosexual behavior since Kinsey's famous survey, no clear explanation of the cause or causes of the homosexual orientation has yet emerged. Older theories about hereditary origins of the condition have not been definitively excluded, but they lack any strong support. If several brothers raised in the same home manifest the orientation it could just as well arise from environmental as from genetic influences.

Dr. Peterson, in the article cited above from the Pope John Center volume *Human Sexuality and Personhood*, speculates about the dual programming for both male and female that exists in every developing human embryo until the sixth week of prégnancy.[10] He notes that a similar duality of sexual development occurs in the brain of the fetus. This might indicate that the hormones program the brain to develop specific kinds of sexual behavior. This could, in theory at least, include a homosexual orientation as hormonally influenced, but little information to support this has yet been found.

There is little evidence to suggest that the typical permanent homosexual orientation is the result of repeated homosexual activity as such. *The preference seems, at least in cases of the permanent orientation, to precede the activity.* It may be that the activity can fix a preference more deeply into the personality of a young person, since research data underscore different strengths of homosexual preference.

The most popular theories about the origins of the homosexual preference still relate it to early psychological development. Sigmund Freud expressed this in 1935 in a letter from Austria to an American mother with a homosexual son: *"We consider it (homosexuality) to be a variation of the sexual function produced by a certain arrest of sexual development."*[11]

Dr. John R. Cavanagh published a thorough study of homosexuality in 1966 entitled *Counseling the Invert.* He revised it in 1977 and added several new chapters plus two chapters by Rev. John Harvey O.S.F.S.[12] Chapters 6 and 7 of that volume review much of the modern speculation about the causes of homosexuality. Dr. Cavanagh himself reaches the conclusion, "Deviant sexuality, including homosexuality, is a result of a personality or character problem in which the sexual orientation of the individual becomes fixated at an early age."[13]

Speculation about what factors might contribute to fixing the homosexual orientation focuses on familial and peer relationships like the distant father factor mentioned already. A boy who is sheltered by his mother from other boys, or who is sickly, may theoretically never develop normal peer relationships, and then may eventually offer himself as a sexual object so as to be accepted and embraced by peers or other males. If he has not identified with his own sex through his father or boy friends, he may identify with a female way of viewing reality.

Other familial factors which may influence homosexual orientation for both males and females include deprivation of normal family life for those living in institutions, anti-sexual puritanism in the home, early unconscious seduction of a child by parents in circumstances of extreme immodesty, and a rigid, loveless family life. Even such factors as a bad case of acne, extreme shyness, or the habit of stammering may influence a boy or girl toward exclusive companionship and affection with his or her own sex.

If these familial factors really do contribute significantly to an eventual permanent homosexual orientation with the incumbent social and moral difficulties it poses, an ounce of prevention may be worth a pound of cure.

Treatment of Homosexual Persons

Treatment of homosexual persons is complex and challenging. Since some social and psychological influences seem commonly to accompany a homosexual orientation, it may even be possible to treat original causes of which homosexual orientation is the manifestation. *Particularly in the case of young persons, it seems important in therapy to focus primarily on the personality problems rather than on the homosexual inclination.*

In his letter to the mother of a homosexual son, Sigmund Freud spoke optimistically of therapy, not primarily for homosexuality, but for the person. "If he is unhappy, neurotic, torn by conflicts, inhibited in his social life," Freud wrote, "analysis may bring him harmony, peace of mind, and full efficiency whether he remains a homosexual or gets changed."[14]

Therapists can deal with sexual compulsion in the human person. A compulsion may be described as a fascination with some object or obedience to an impulse accompanied by the conviction, based on previous

167

experience, that the particular fascination or impulse is irresistible. While some homosexual persons may have as much control over their tendencies as the average heterosexual person, others may be as compulsive as alcoholics. The compulsive nature of some homosexual behavior may be inferred from the squalid surroundings where the acts sometimes occur, such as in public toilets, coupled with the risk of recrimination and disease.

Can treatment overcome a person's homosexual orientation and replace it with a heterosexual one? It seems clear that this can never happen without the person's own deep desire and profound commitment to change. The most likely cases of change of orientation can be expected where the homosexual orientation was not deeply rooted or completely exclusive of heterosexual interest.

W. H. Masters and V. E. Johnson of St. Louis, Missouri, in 1979 reported significant success in changing homosexual orientation.[15] However, the majority of the 67 persons in their program had prior heterosexual experience and two-thirds were married. Professionals in the field have great reservations about the consistent success of either psychoanalytic or behavioral efforts to change a permanent and exclusive homosexual orientation.[16]

On the other hand, a trend has developed among some therapists, motivated in part by pressures from homosexual organizations, to focus treatment of homosexual persons on the enhancement of their homosexual functioning instead of changing their orientation.[17] Thus, some counselors have begun using marriage counseling techniques with homosexual couples who are living together. Others have attempted to reduce specific sexual dysfunction such as impotence and premature ejaculation.

The moral ideals of the Judeo-Christian tradition and Catholic teaching to be reviewed in the next chapter will raise serious moral objections to the use of therapy to enhance homosexual activity. However, therapeutic counseling can benefit some homosexual persons, regarding both the special difficulties they often experience in social relationships, and also, as with heterosexual persons as well, in developing their own self-esteem and mature character formation. Therapy and pastoral counseling can assist homosexual persons to avoid homosexual activity and the situations which foster it.

In the light of many comparative studies of homosexual and heterosexual persons, it seems fair to say that homosexual orientation itself is not clearly linked with some psychological abnormality.[18] Since exclusive homosexual preference represents such a statistical minority (4% of the male population), it would seem fair also to say that special factors are necessary for its development, but no research to date has been able to delineate those factors. In any case, those persons who are homosexual are faced with challenges unparalleled in the heterosexual world. The next chapter will explore those challenges, particularly the challenge of forming chaste relationships with both heterosexual and homosexual persons.

Discussion Questions

1. Why does this chapter not speak simply and concisely about "homo-sexuals?"
2. What did the Saghir and Robbins study discover about persons of homosexual orientation?
3. Can a person engage in heterosexual activities while entertaining homosexual fantasies? Can you cite the case mentioned above?
4. What suggestion can be made to improve on the Kinsey Scale of sexual preference?
5. What do the most popular theories about the origin of the homo-sexual orientation suggest as the cause?
6. What new trend has developed among some therapists for their care of homosexual persons? Does this trend conform to Catholic teach-ing?

Notes

1. Karlen, Arlo, *Sexuality and Homosexuality* (N.Y., N.Y., W. W. Norton Co., 1971).

2. Pauly, I. and Goldstein, S., "Physicians' Attitudes in Treating Homosexuals," *Medical Aspects of Human Sexuality*, 1970, 4:26–45.

3. Bell, Alan P., "The Homosexual as Patient," in *Human Sexuality*, edited by Richard Green M.D., 2nd edit. (Baltimore, MD, Williams & Wilkins Co., 1979), pp. 98–114.

4. Reprinted in *Human Sexuality and Personhood* (St. Louis, MO, The Pope John Center, 1981), pp. 91–93.

5. Saghir, M. P., and Robbins, E., *Male and Female Homosexuality* (Baltimore, MD, Williams & Wilkins Co., 1973).

6. Hooker, Evelyn, "Male Homosexuals and Their 'Worlds'," in *Sexual Inversion*, edited by Judd Marmor (N.Y., N.Y.: Basic Books Inc., 1965), pp. 83–107 at p. 86.

7. Ovesey, Lionel, "Pseudohomosexuality and Homosexuality in Men: Psychodynamics as a Guide to Treatment" in *Sexual Inversion, op. cit.*, pp. 211–231.

8. Peterson, Rev. Michael R., "Psychological Aspects of Human Sexual Behaviors" in *Human Sexuality and Personhood, op. cit.*, pp. 86–110, at pp. 89–91.

9. *Ibid.*, pp. 90–91.

10. *Ibid.*, pp. 96–109.

11. Cf. Cavanagh, John R., *Counseling the Homosexual* (Huntington, IN, Our Sunday Visitor, Inc., 1977), p. 248.

12. *Ibid.*

13. *Ibid.*, p. 58.

14. *Ibid.*, p. 248.

15. Masters, W. H., and Johnson, V. E., *Homosexuality in Perspective* (Boston: Little, Brown and Co., 1979).

16. Coleman, Eli, "Changing Approaches to the Treatment of Homosexuality," *American Behavioral Scientist*, 25:4, Mar. 1 Op. 1982, pp. 397–400.

17. *Ibid.*, pp. 401–405.

18. Bell, *op.cit.*, pp. 112–113.

Preview of Chapter Fifteen

● Homosexual persons are often unfairly judged according to various stereotypes, these social myths create a kind of imprisonment.

● Overcoming these stereotypes does not mean that homosexual activity becomes morally right and good.

● The morality of homosexual behavior should be judged on the basis of the inherent meaning and purpose of human genital sexuality, its essential and indispensable finality.

● Homosexual activity lacks this finality; it does not accord with the Biblical norm and ideals for human sexuality.

● Church teaching does not accept moral justification for homosexual acts on the grounds that they would be consonant with the condition of such people.

● The deeper need of any human is for friendship, rather than genital expression.

C H A P T E R 15

Moral Guidance for Homosexuals

In their essay on the training of priests the Fathers of the Second Vatican Council urged the cultivation of aptitudes which are "most conducive to dialogue" and of the "willingness to listen to others and the capacity to open their hears in a spirit of charity to the various needs of their fellow men."[1]

Anyone who would offer moral guidance to homosexuals must possess these qualities in abundance. Even after a concerted effort, a non-homosexual person can only begin to grasp the full impact of the stigma society has traditionally attached to homosexuals.

Consider four of the *stereotypes widely accepted by non-homosexuals* as applying to all persons with a homosexual orientation:

- that all homosexuals are attracted to children and adolescents and wish to have physical contact with them.

- that all male homosexuals are effeminate and lack of typical male characteristics of courage, aggressiveness, and strength.

- that all homosexuals are sexually active.

- that all homosexuals can change their orientation merely by willing to do so and by cultivating heterosexual friendships.

Adding up these four stereotypes produces an incorrect and unfair image of all homosexual persons, yet one which is, unfortunately, still commonly accepted by many heterosexual persons. Furthermore, the fact that individual homosexuals themselves know the image is false does not adequately protect them from the stigma it fosters.

The term "coming out of the closet" designates the action of a homosexual who publicly announces his or her homosexual orientation. It also indicates that *homosexuals experience a kind of imprisonment* because of the social myths which surround them.

Homosexuals are a minority and have a different sexual orientation from the majority of people, so they suffer the same problems as all minority groups. In addition, they usually keep their membership in this minority a secret. They must constantly avoid arousing suspicion of their true identity. Blackmailers often seek to capitalize on the threat of revealing a homosexual's secret. Obviously such difficulties are reduced if the homosexual person does not engage in homosexual activity.

Yet heterosexual persons seldom experience the alienation that homosexuals endure. Hiding their true identities in a mixed society, homosexuals cannot help but feel like strangers. In a society that makes cruel jokes about "fags" and "queers" they may suffer a tremendous loneliness and lack of self-esteem. Many homosexuals assimilate the horror that society manifests toward them and consciously or unconsciously hate themselves.

Hence, persons anxious to offer moral guidance to homosexual persons must first heed the Indian proverb, "Before judging someone, first walk a mile in his moccasins." The stigma which society has attached to homosexual persons seems with increasing clarity to be an immoral response to a deeply troubled minority within society. *This does not, of course, mean that homosexual activity becomes morally right and good.*

In their zeal for erasing the unjust stigma attached to homosexuals, some scholars and writers have taken just such a position. They have argued that homosexuality should be seen as a natural and morally equivalent alternative to heterosexuality. Some would even go farther and argue that in an overpopulated world it is morally preferable, or at least justifiable as contraception. A favorite analogy proposes that homosexual activity is no more immoral than writing left-handed instead of right-handed.

Morality of Homosexual Activity

Undoubtedly some members of the American Psychiatric Association reflected this view of moral neutrality in their controversial vote on Dec. 15, 1973, to remove homosexuality from the status of a pathological condition in their diagnostic manual. But the psychological evaluation of homosexual behavior should not be confused with the evaluation of its morality.

In the light of the stigma society has attached to homosexual persons and the self-hatred this stigma engenders, one might expect homosexual persons to manifest pathological personality profiles. *The fact that many do not reflects to their credit, not society's.*

But many persons who perform obviously immoral actions may be perfectly normal in their psychological profile. Hence, the fact that homosexual activity may not be a definite symptom of mental disease or of a psychologically abnormal personality tells nothing about the morality of such activity.

The spontaneous and habitual quality of the sexual behavior of homosexual persons offers no indication whatsoever that such behavior is *morally* good or even morally neutral. For instance, a left-handed preference in writing or throwing a baseball *is* morally neutral. But gluttony, excessive drinking, continual lying, and non-therapeutic use of drugs may also be spontaneous and habitual, yet such behavior is clearly *not morally neutral.* Kleptomania, defined as a persistent neurotic impulse to steal, especially without economic motive, might be called a habitual and spontaneous preference for objectively immoral behavior.

The question homosexual persons are asking is, "Why does society generally consider our sexual behavior immoral when for us it seems perfectly harmless and fulfilling?"

As a matter of fact, American society has become more and more accepting of homosexual behavior. Activists in the gay rights movement have sponsored demonstrations to support their "rights" to homosexual activity. Legal experts are beginning to describe homosexual activity between consenting adults as "victimless," and hence not a criminal activity.

Crimes like murder, stealing, rape and abduction can easily be classified as immoral behavior because they immediately attack the common good and the rights of other persons. But this reasoning does not apply with such immediacy to homosexual activity between consenting adults. Nor does it so readily apply, incidentally, to heterosexual activity between unmarried but consenting adults. In the long run both kinds of activity may weaken the stability of marriage and family life, but this cannot easily be documented.

In any case, while the legal status of homosexual behavior may depend primarily on whether it immediately affects the common good or the rights of others, these concerns are not the primary basis for its moral analysis. *The morality of homosexual behavior must be evaluated in the light of the inherent meaning and purpose of genital activity.*

The traditional designation of homosexual activity as a *perversion* indicated it was activity turned against what is right and good. Some authors are using the term *inversion* which does not include the notion of the right and good, but simply denotes a reversal from heterosexual to homosexual activity.

Hence the controversy over the moral significance of homosexual behavior boils down to asking whether homosexual genital activity violates the meaning and purpose of genital activity itself. If it does, the fact that persons of a homosexual orientation find it desirable will not make it morally acceptable.

Previous discussions in this volume have supported the view that the inherent meaning of genital activity is found in its capacity to express a totally unifying and generously procreating relationship—the covenant of marriage. This inherent meaning or purpose of genital activity can be called its *finality.*

Thus the "Declaration on Certain Questions Concerning Sexual Ethics" of the Vatican Congregation for the Doctrine of the Faith gave a succinct judgment on homosexual activity: *"For according to the objective moral order, homosexual relations are acts which lack an essential and indispensable finality."*[2]

This evaluation of homosexual activity as violating the moral order and the authentic finality of human genital activity has been strongly supported in the Judeo-Christian tradition and taught with the authority of the Catholic magisterium. But is has been questioned and challenged from a variety of perspectives. For example, the Biblical texts which oppose homosexual behavior have been questioned.

Biblical Teaching on Homosexuality

Both Old and New Testament passages explicitly oppose homosexual activity. For example, two Old Testament passages (Lev. 18:22 and 20:13) strongly condemn the "abomination" of homosexual behavior. Some critics have alleged that these condemnations depend on the connection of such behavior with pagan cultic activity. Scholars like Joseph Jensen O.S.B. have strongly objected to such an interpretation.[3]

The New Testament passages condemning homosexual behavior are found in Romans 1:24 24–28, I Cor. 6:9–10, and I Tim. 1:9–10. The

175

clearest reference is Romans 1:26–27: "God therefore delivered them up to shameful passions. Their woman exchanged natural intercourse for unnatural, and the men gave up natural intercourse with women and burned with lust for one another. Men did shameful things with men, and thus received in their own persons the penalty for their perversity."

Some critics have alleged that the condemnation by St. Paul is limited to homosexual activity by those with a heterosexual orientation. Others have suggested that St. Paul was more concerned that the pagans had abandoned God than with the consequences (homosexual behavior) of this abandonment.

It is quite possible that St. Paul and the people of ancient times knew little about a homosexual personality orientation. What is not proven is that this knowledge would have made a difference. *The Pauline texts condemn a kind of human activity which does not accord with the Biblical norm and ideals for human sexuality.*

The fact that St. Paul in Romans, Chapter 1, is primarily concerned with opposing idolatry indicates no lack of concern for homosexual activity. The opposite seems to be true. The homosexual activity reveals what St. Paul calls a "depraved sense," the result of abandoning God. Paul makes the Roman Christians conscious of the evil of idolatry by appealing to an evil they were well aware of, the depravity of the pagans' conduct. If the conduct was not considered depraved, the argument would have been meaningless.

It would be a mistake to suppose that the Biblical teaching on homosexuality is confined to the few explicit texts just mentioned. The Biblical teaching on sexuality reviewed above in Chapter One stresses the complementary relationship of man and woman and the twofold unitive/procreative meaning of marriage. Nowhere is there any approval of homosexual unions, whereas heterosexual marriage is confirmed from *Genesis* to *Revelation*. The continuous and firm judgment of Catholic teaching which considers homosexual activity immoral is *rooted in this Biblical heritage* and its understanding of the human person and human sexuality.

Theories of Compromise

A second kind of challenge to Catholic teaching on the immorality of homosexual activity comes from those who recognize heterosexuality as the ideal and norm but wish to make exceptions based on the circumstances of some homosexual relationships. Some authors, for example, say that in an ideal world homosexuality would be wrong, but given the sinful world in which we live, it can be morally acceptable, at least in stable, loving relationships comparable to marriage.

The justification of homosexuality because of sin in the world suggests a possible comparison with the use of force to combat aggression. Force or violence would be wrong except for the fact that there is sinful aggression in the world. In this sense, sufficient violence is permissible as is necessary to cope with unjust aggression. But one cannot draw a parallel to homosexuality. Even if a person's homosexual orientation were judged to be the result of sin in the world, coping with it would demand resistance rather than capitulation.

In fact, traditional Catholic teaching regards as immoral, not homosexual *orientation*, but *homosexual activity*. Hence the question of sin hinges on human freedom while performing human actions. The person who freely chooses homosexual behavior sins, whereas any non-free homosexual acts are not sinful, though objectively immoral.

The theory of ethical proportionalism discussed earlier in this volume has been invoked by some authors in support of a compromise theory on homosexuality. They would prosper that in some situations what they call the *"ontic"* or *"premoral"* evil because in these situations a favorable proportion of good in reference to evil will be found. The proportion is to be located in the judgment that excusing factors and positive values counterbalance the presumed evil of the acts.

The most obvious practical objection to this approach is the problem of weighing the excusing factors. Those persons who are advised that homosexual activity is morally acceptable for them in given circumstances are implicitly told that a judgment has been made which favors this activity. Who can make such a judgment and on what basis? How long does it remain valid? How does it account for freedom and grace?

On a theoretical level, moreover, proportionalism seems here to bypass the relationship of acts to persons. if *homosexual acts are contrary to a person's own bodily sexual nature and the goal of one's moral life, one cannot logically assume that they contain only "ontic" or "premoral" evil.* And if they involve moral evil, no amount of circumstances can neutralize that fact.

The Vatican "Declaration on Certain Questions Concerning Sexual Ethics" mentioned above excludes explicitly the use of a theory of compromise or ethical proportionalism in providing moral guidance to homosexuals. It addresses the problem of confirmed homosexual persons who feel incapable of enduring a solitary life and who pursue homosexual relations within a sincere communion of life and love analogous to marriage.

The Declaration recognizes that subjective moral guilt may be reduced and points out that "culpability will be judged with prudence in such cases." But, in terms of a moral analysis, it adds explicitly, "No pastoral method can be employed which would give moral justification to these acts on the grounds that they would be consonant with the condition of such people."[4]

A Vatican Letter to the Bishops of the World

Despite the clarity of the Vatican Declaration, a number of groups continued and even intensified pressure to have Catholic teaching on this issue reversed. In response, Vatican officials with the express approval of Pope John Paul II issued a letter in 1986 to the Catholic Bishops of the world: The Pastoral Care of Homosexual Persons.[5] It reiterated the basic equality and dignity of homosexual persons with all other human beings, and condemned absolutely any speech or action which violates homosexual persons' rights to acceptance and friendship within both the Church and society at large. Most fundamentally, the Letter defended their right to be free of violence in word or act. At the same time, it warned that efforts to seek civil recognition for homosexual actions or pairing (as legally on a par with heterosexual acts or marriage) is likely to incite unstable persons to serious violations of even the true rights of homosexual persons.

The document also pointed out that homosexual persons, like all other human beings, must face the fact that they too limp morally. For we all have things within us at least certain tendencies which we can rightly call "objective disorders." These are tendencies which in *objective* reality pull us towards *disordered* acts which can damage and even destroy us and others. For any individual, these tendencies might include strong, habitual tendencies towards, for instance, conceit, or greed, or drunkenness, or angry rage, or laziness. For many, and perhaps most, heterosexual persons they include also tendencies towards sexual disorders: masturbation, fornication, adultery, voyeurism, etc. Any one of these "objectively disordered" tendencies can cause each of us to limp morally, to get through life in an upright way only with great interior struggle. To have these tendencies is not itself a sin, but, sadly, at times, these tendencies contribute perhaps even to one's failing in a serious way morally. Homosexual persons, the Letter notes, cannot claim exemption from the struggle against such tendencies. Indeed, an honest desire for the truth will lead all to recognize that the homosexual tendency is itself one type of "objective disorder."

In the discussion which followed the publication of the declaration . . . an overly benign interpretation was given to the homosexual condition itself, some going so far as to call it neutral or even good. Although the particular inclination of the homosexual person is not sin, it is a more or less strong tendency ordered toward an intrinsic moral evil and thus the inclination itself must be seen as an objective disorder.[6]

In this, then, as well as in all else, the homosexual person is like the rest of us. Indeed certain other persons in this world suffer and struggle morally more than homosexual persons or the generality of the rest of mankind do. No theory of compromise of the type mentioned above can exempt the homosexual person from his or her particular kind of moral struggle.

Underlying the theory of compromise about the morality of homosexual acts is the seemingly overwhelming challenge most persons, homosexuals included, face in remaining celibate. There is good reasons to hold that one cannot lead a celibate life over a long period of time on his own resources. It will not be easy, even with the help of God.

Yet, homosexual persons are not the only persons, other than religious under vows, called to a life of celibacy. Although celibacy may be chosen in support of an ideal, "for the sake of the kingdom of heaven," the New Testament personalism described in Chapter One presents the option of celibacy as a way of life to which anyone may be called. The call to celibacy would seem to be given, according to the Church teaching, not only to homosexual persons, but to divorced persons and to persons for whom marriage is not possible. The latter group includes those persons mentally or physically or psychologically unable to marry as well as those who simply have no realistic hopes of finding a suitable partner for marriage.

Like all of us, too, homosexual persons can win out in this struggle only to the extent that they work with God's grace, that is, the healing and truth which God offers each human being is his or her innermost mind and heart. For Christians, this means more and more consciously seeking the friendship of Jesus Christ. It means, too, accepting the respect and support which God gives each of us in our brothers and sisters in the Faith. For Catholic homosexual persons, this means especially accepting the friendship, encouragement, guidance, and, if needed at times, the forgiveness which the whole Church and her Lord extend to us in the absolution of a priest. And, though the Letter does not mention it, the Church encourages Catholic homosexuals to band together in support groups which promote celibate chastity as the only acceptable goal for any homosexual person, and provide the companionship and spiritual direction to make it a reality.

Particular Problems of Homosexuals

Homosexual persons, however, face additional problems in attempting to remain celibate. The stigma which society attaches to homosexuality and the alienation this fosters drives homosexual persons to seek security and dignity in relationships with other homosexuals. The theory that homosexual activity is morally neutral like left-handedness offers encouragement to adopt a life-style which features homosexual "dating" and "marriage."

The response of the Church to these problems is that she cannot condone this life-style and cannot approve the activist organizations which seem to encourage it among young homosexuals. *But the Church can reach out to offer homosexual persons respect, friendship, and justice.* She can love homosexual persons as members of the Body of Christ even as she calls them to sublimate the sexual energy which leads to homosexual activity.

The U.S. Bishops in writing of homosexuals and their needs in a pastoral reflection on the moral life in 1976 concluded with an appeal for "a special degree of pastoral understanding and care."[7]

The U.S. Bishops Committee on Pastoral Research and Practices in 1973 published a booklet of *Principles to Guide Confessors in Questions of Homosexuality.*[8] It speaks of instances where a homosexual person seeks to break out of the homosexual environment. Such individuals need motivation and encouragement to leave this environment which provided some measure of human affection and acceptance. This challenge to the homosexual accentuates the need for heterosexual persons who will also offer affection and acceptance. *"The deeper need of any human is for friendship rather than genital expression,"* according to this document, and homosexuals "should seek to form stable friendships among both homosexuals and heterosexuals."

This statement also suggests that "a homosexual can have an abiding relationship with another homosexual without genital expression." But it adds the caution that, "If the relationship, however, has reached a stage where the homosexual is not able to avoid overt actions, he should be admonished to break off the relationship."

In addressing confessors this document recommends that homosexuals can live chastely in the world with the help of regular spiritual direction, a plan of life including prayer, the sacraments, and some specific work of charity, and at least one stable friendship.

Since October, 1980, a group called "Courage" has been meeting weekly in New York to carry out this very program.⁹ Members gather to foster a spirit of fellowship and to ensure that individuals will not have to face the problems of homosexuality alone. They believe that chaste friendships are not only possible but necessary in celibate Christian life. Through "Courage" they are able to obtain spiritual direction and guidance in a plan of spiritual life. They recognize that alone they are powerless to lead a spiritually and humanly satisfying life, but can do so in the group and with the grace of God, working through the group.

This admission closely parallels the first of the 12 steps of Alcoholics Anonymous. One retreat director who presents a special retreat for homosexual persons begins with this very similarity. It raises useful comparisons to an area of nonsexual behavior where persons also experience some forms of addiction and compulsion.

The AA therapy of abstinence parallels closely the pastoral advice which Church teaching offers homosexuals regarding genital activity. Alcoholics who give up "social drinking" are not expected to give up social relationships, but to dispense with alcohol. Homosexuals are not expected to give up social relationships either, but they can dispense with genital activity.

One of the problems facing homosexuals in the United States is that of the spread of AIDS (acquired immune deficiency syndrome). AIDS is at present an incurable disease. It is transmitted through intimate sexual contact, contact with contaminated blood or other body fluids, or through organ donation; it can be transmitted to children by a mother during pregnancy or parturition. Approximately 25% of persons with AIDS in the United States are drug users who have employed contaminated needles or other drug equipment.

However, currently about two-thirds of AIDS victims in the country are homosexual or bisexual men. U.S. government education programs concerning AIDS prevention have encouraged the use of condoms by both heterosexuals and homosexuals as a way of "safe sex". Yet, the Catholic bishops have indicated

"So-called 'safe sex' practices are at best only partially effective. They do not take into account either the real values that are at stake or the fundamental good of the human person. . . . The best approach to the prevention of AIDS ought to be based on the communication of a value-centered understanding of the meaning of human personhood. . . , the importance of chastity, and the power of God's love which enables us to live a chaste life" ("The Many Faces of AIDS: A Gospel Response", USCC Admin. Board, *Origins*, Dec. 24, 1987, pp. 486–7).

Moral Growth and Development

This discussion has focused primarily on the moral evaluation of homosexual activity. Some contemporary authors and counselors have shifted their attention to overlook these actions and focus on the attitudes and motivation of the persons who engage in homosexual activity. This shift in focus helps to distinguish a wide variety of homosexual relationships ranging from forms of prostitution through chance encounters to tender and unselfish relationships. This range parallels heterosexual relationships which take similar forms. But in heterosexual relationships the range climaxes with the ideal and enduring relationship of marriage which offers personal fulfillment and a Sacramental covenant to reflect in the world Christ's sacrificial love for the Church.

Those whose moral reflection overlooks actions in favor of persons tend to encourage the formation of permanent homosexual relationships modeled on heterosexual marriage. Clearly such relationships are in less contradiction to the dignity of persons and the Christian vocation of love than are the furtive homosexual encounters of near strangers.

But a radical objection remains. Human persons are bodily creatures and cannot detach themselves from corporeal nature. If the homosexual genital activity of the body contradicts sexual activity's own inherent purpose and meaning, *the psychic predisposition and loving intention of a person cannot superimpose a different authentic meaning on the genital activity*. If it could, the human person would not genuinely be an incarnate being with interdependent body and spirit. Rather the human person would become an autonomous, independent spirit, divorced from the body and able to manipulate it as a pottery-maker molds clay.

Hence the profound challenge which faces homosexual persons calls for their developing interpersonal relationships while respecting the moral objections to pursuing such relationships to the point of genital expression. The gift of human freedom entitles persons to direct their bodily activities in accord with moral convictions and the norms of authentic love. But the freedom of homosexuals to direct their behavior must confront radical difficulties because of loneliness, social alienation, and their own psychological dispositions.

Moral growth, in this context, means the basic human process of integrating one's impulses and sexual passions in accord with the ideals

182

of authentic love and good judgment. Such a process takes a lifetime for everyone, although homosexual persons will experience vividly the frustration which their unusual personality orientation engenders. But the concluding word of moral guidance to homosexual persons should be the hopeful and encouraging promise of St. Augustine based on the redeeming grace of Jesus Christ:

> *God does not command the impossible, but in commanding advises you to do what you can and to pray for help to do what may seem impossible, and he gives you the help to make it possible.*[10]

Discussion Questions

1. What four stereotypes help create a false image of homosexual persons?
2. What basis does this discussion offer for evaluating the morality of homosexual behavior?
3. What does Biblical teaching say about homosexual activity?
4. What basis can you offer for saying that the evil in homosexual activity is not merely ontic or premoral evil?
5. Why is the deeper need of any human for friendship rather than genital expression?
6. What points of similarity can you find between persons seeking to avoid homosexual activity and persons joining Alcoholic Anonymous?

Notes

1. *On the Training of Priests (Optatam Totius)*, in *Vatican Council II, The Conciliar and Post Conciliar Documents*, ed. by Austin Flannery O.P. (Collegeville, MN: The Liturgical Press), #16.
2. Published December 29, 1975, #8.
3. *Human Sexuality and Personhood*, (St. Louis, MO, The Pope John Center, 1981), pp. 23–26.
4. #8.
5. *Origins*, November 13, 1986, vol. 16: no. 22, pp. 377–382.
6. *Ibid., p. 379.*
7. "To Live in Christ Jesus," Nov. 11, 1976, Washington, D.C., The U.S. Catholic Conference, p. 19.
8. Washington, D.C., The U.S. Catholic Conference, p. 11.
9. For information, contact:

Fr. John Harvey OSFS, c/o *Courage*, P.O. Box 913,
Old Chelsea Station, New York, NY 10113
Phone (212) 421–0426.

10. *De Natura et Gratia*, c. 43. #50 (CSEL 60,270).

Preview of
Chapter Sixteen

● Infertility, a great burden to many married couples, can be treated in many cases by administration of hormones, by standard surgical repair, or by microsurgery.

● Artificial insemination of the husband's sperm has only succeeded in 15–20% of couples using it because of poor semen quality from the husband.

● Artificial insemination from a donor creates the problem of whether to inform the child later in addition to serious moral objections.

● *In vitro* fertilization brings together the male sperm and the female ovum in a Petri dish and then implants the very young embryo in the woman's uterus.

● Surrogate parenting uses reproductive technology so that a woman carries a child throughout pregnancy but relinquishes it after birth.

CHAPTER 16

Technological Reproduction of Human Persons

Introduction

About ten to fifteen percent of all married couples in the United States and Canada are infertile, while an additional ten percent have fewer children than they wish. Couples who are involuntarily childless can find this experience to be a great burden which sometimes leads to the breakdown of a marriage or, in extreme cases, even to suicide. *Until fairly recent times there was not much that could be done about curing or correcting infertility.* It was thought that the infertility was due to the woman, and so some husbands would seek other women and marry them to obtain the child they desired.

An Englishman, Dr. John Hunter (1728–1793), and a contemporary French physician, Professor Thouret, were both credited with the first successful attempts to bring about artificial insemination. This was done in the late 1700s following developments in animal husbandry. The technique generally was not picked up by the other practitioners and the procedure went into hiding. It was not until about 1865 that medical journals began to report an increasing use of artificial insemination.

From then until the late 1970s there was no other technological means available to help the infertile couple besides artificial insemination. However, in 1978 on July 25, a baby girl, Louise Brown, was born in England. She was the first child successfully to be conceived in a "test tube" and be safely delivered. Since that date the use of *in vitro* fertilization to obtain a conception has increased rapidly.

The Problem of Infertility

Definition

A convenient way to define human infertility is to say it is the condition of a couple who, having had regular intercourse without the use of any contraception for one year, have not achieved a pregnancy.

Causes of Infertility—Female Factors

There are a number of factors in women that may result in infertility. Among these are: the failure of ovulation, endometriosis, allergy to sperm, a build up of antibodies in the female genital tract causing the sperm to clump together and to thus render them useless for fertilization, closed fallopian tubes due to infection or accident, and certain sterilizing operations. Other causes of female infertility are congenital malformations, tumors of the pituitary, and cervical factors such as infection or the inadequate production of cervical mucus.

Causes of Infertility—Male Factors

Causes of male infertility include diabetes which may result in impotence; endocrine failures so that sperm production is inhibited; obstruction of the sperm duct due to injury or infection or sterilizing operations; and failure of the semen to liquefy in the vaginal tract, thus keeping them from traveling through the cervix. Another major cause of male infertility is the production of abnormal semen. This condition can come from a high bodily temperature, tight-fitting clothing, hot baths, or even prolonged sitting!

Impact of Infertility

On a nationwide scale the problem is not small. A published survey reported that in the past 20 years or so, some 250,000 children have been born as a result of artificial insemination. The annual rate is somewhere between 6,000 and 10,000.

For the couples who slowly realize that they are infertile it is very difficult to accept the fact that they cannot give each other a child who is biologically related to both of them. The child was supposed to symbolize their mutual love, be a constant witness to it. *Consequently, if they discover a means to overcome this severe life-crisis, they will welcome it enthusiastically.* In some instances, the couple is mutually willing to accept the biological contribution of a third party so as to ensure that they can have a child who is biologically related to at least one of them. For this option to be successful, their inability to have a child together and the pain it evoked need to be accepted and integrated by each.

Treatment of Infertility

In view of the large variety of causes of infertility in one or other of the spouses, it is necessary first of all that an appropriate diagnostic evaluation take place. Once the source of the infertility is determined, the appropriate measures can be instituted. *These measures may include the administration of hormones, standard surgical repair, or the modern techniques of microsurgery.* Microsurgery is used more commonly in the reversal of vasectomies and tubal ligations. Yet, in spite of all the information available and the development of new correcting techniques, there remain some individuals who cannot be helped by these procedures. It is for these individuals that some of the new reproductive technologies have been developed.

This chapter will present a brief overview of these technologies. The following chapter will consider the morality of technological reproduction.

Reproductive Technologies

Definition

By the term reproductive technologies we mean those procedures which have been devised to assist a couple to have a child. This does *not* necessarily mean that the wife will contribute the egg and the husband the sperm, because one or both can be obtained from other human persons. The reproductive technologies covered in this chapter will be artificial insemination (AI), *in vitro* fertilization (IVF), embryo transplantation (ET) and surrogate parenting.

187

Types of Reproductive Technologies

Artificial Insemination. Artificial insemination using the husband's sperm (AIH) is ordinarily performed 1) when the quality of the semen is poor due to a reduced sperm concentration or a very small volume of semen, and 2) when, although the semen is good, there are an insufficient number of sperm present in the cervical mucus. Usually, AIH is performed two or three times at mid-cycle in order to bracket the time of ovulation. A semen sample is obtained by masturbation into a sterile container, after which it is inserted through the vagina and deposited usually at the mouth of the cervix. *The results of AIH have not been too good; perhaps only 15–20 percent of couples trying it for reasons of poor semen quality actually achieved pregnancy.*

Artificial insemination with donor semen has been used in cases where the husband's semen simply is not capable of bringing on a pregnancy. This may occur when the sperm count is very low or the sperm are lifeless. The technique is basically the same as in AIH except that the semen is obtained from some other individual. Medical students are a common source of such semen. The presumption is that they offer a high grade source of semen. Ideally, the donor should be of the same racial stock and bear some physical resemblance to the "presumed father." Furthermore, some sort of genetic screening is now being urged so as to lessen the possibility of mating two carriers of a serious genetic disorder.

Generally, the donor and the couple are unknown to each other. There is no generally accepted rule as to informing the child later that he or she is the product of artificial insemination with donor sperm. On the basis of experience with adopted children, some advocate that the child be informed when old enough to comprehend the message.

In both cases (husband and donor sources), frozen semen can be used, although more frequently it is the donor semen that is frozen. The semen may be kept frozen for several years without damage or apparent loss of power. It is calculated that there have been some 10,000 births in the United States that resulted from the use of frozen semen.

In Vitro Fertilization (IVF). The basic procedure of this technology is the obtaining of the semen from the husband by masturbation as one would for artificial insemination, while the egg is obtained from the wife by means of laparoscopy. The egg and sperm are brought together in a Petri dish where a sperm fertilizes the egg. After several cell divisions, the young embryo is placed into the wife's uterus where, if all goes well, it implants in a few days and proceeds to develop as normal.

IVF—Informed Consent. Before a couple enters an IVF program they should be thoroughly informed of all its aspects. The husband and wife

188

are requested to sign an informed consent form which contains at least the following items:

1. A description of reasonably anticipated risks
2. A clear statement that a successful conception, pregnancy or birth is *not* guaranteed
3. An acknowledgement that malformations of the infant are possible
4. A description of available prenatal diagnostic procedures.

IVF—The Method. The obtaining of the egg from the wife is a process which requires careful timing. The details of the procedure and its timing were investigated thoroughly by British researchers, among others, Dr. Robert Edwards and Dr. Richard Steptoe, as well as by groups in Australia and elsewhere.

The woman's cycle is followed carefully and at the appropriate time a hormone or a fertility pill is given to bring about superovulation. This means that several eggs mature about the same time and can be collected together. Inducing ovulation in this way has the advantage of being able to set and accurately predict the time of ovulation. This control allows for good planning and integration of the other activities necessary to the procedure.

Furthermore, the obtaining of several eggs at the same time from the one woman allows two or more embryos to be produced. Replacement of multiple embryos into the woman's uterus increases the chance that at least one will implant. Of course, the possibility of twins or triplets should not be overlooked, *nor should the fact that this procedure may also result in a large number of human embryos being lost.*

After an appropriate number of hours have elapsed, the egg(s) are collected. This is accomplished by the use of the laparoscope, a tube-like instrument which is inserted in the abdomen of the woman. Through the use of fiberoptics it is possible to illuminate the interior of the woman's abdominal cavity and to observe directly the surface of the ovary. When the egg is about to be released, it protrudes from the surface of the ovary somewhat like a blister. With the help of another large needle inserted into the abdomen, the egg is removed by suction and placed into a receptacle containing suitable nutrient fluid.

The container with the egg is transferred from the delivery room to a laboratory where the egg is examined under a microscope. If more than one egg has been collected, each one is placed independently into a drop of semen which is suspended in a small volume of sterile mineral oil. The egg and sperm are allowed to interact for some 10 to 12 hours. At the end of that time, the egg is evaluated by direct microscopic examination to determine whether or not fertilization has taken place. If it

189

has, then the resulting fertilized egg (now called the "zygote") is transferred to another medium which allows the zygote to continue dividing. After several cell divisions, the individual, now an embryo of 6 or 8 cells, is about 2–2½ days of age.

The developing embryo is examined to determine whether its appearance and rate of cell division fall within the normal range. If they do, the embryo is ready for the next step, to be "replaced" in the woman's uterus. Although pregnancies have followed after the transfer of embryos of as few as one cell and as many as sixteen, the most common procedure seems to involve two to eight cell embryos.

Embryo Transfer (ET)

By means of a small diameter Teflon catheter passed through the cervix, the tiny embryo suspended in a minute amount of fluid is transferred into the uterus and deposited carefully at the top of the uterine cavity. The procedure must be done gently without causing pain or bleeding. Experience has shown that when these occur, the chances of a successful pregnancy are lessened. If all goes well, the young embryo implants in the wall of the uterus after several days and its development follows its habitual course.

Recent data concerning IVF success rates in the United States came from 41 fertility clinics that treated 3005 patients in 1986. In these clinics, 4867 stimulation cycles were undertaken, from which 2864 embryo transfers resulted. The number of clinical pregnancies from these transfers was 485. Of these pregnancies, 311 live births occurred—about 11% of embryo transfers. At the more expert programs at some clinics, the success rate of live births from embryo transfers was a bit higher—about 15%. (See: National IVF/ET Registry, *Fertility and Sterility*, 49: 212–215, 1988).

The low rate of IVF embryos brought to actual successful birth, however, has led increasingly to the practice of fertilizing 5 or more ova in vitro, and implanting them all in the uterus. The theory is that this will increase by 5 times the chance that one will survive to birth. Unfortunately, if the pregnancy is allowed to continue this way, it is likely that all five will die before birth. Also few women resorting to IVF are willing to be presented with quintuplets at the end of the process. Around the end of the first trimester, therefore, the attending physician determines which (usually two) are "more advantageously placed" in the uterus. He then "reduces" the pregnancies by killing the remaining embryos, e.g., by inserting through the uterine wall and into the chest of each targeted embryo a needle containing potassium chloride. The injection stops their hearts.

At the present time, many fertility clinics in the United States are freezing embryos at very low temperatures and maintaining them in this state until the woman's cycle is appropriate for receiving implanted embryos. Theoretically, young frozen embryos can be kept for years in this state before thawing and implantation.

This process (called "cryopreservation") raises serious ethical and legal issues, among which are the questions of respect for human life, the risks to the embryo in undergoing the rigors of freezing and thawing, the disposing of unwanted embryos, and the relationship of the frozen embryos to their parents. In fertility centers around the country, hundreds of frozen embryos are in storage. Some couples will not use their extra embryos because of the success they have had with first implantation. For other embryos, their parents will have died before implantation, become divorced or disabled, or simply decide for various reasons (e.g. because of financial or psychological factors) that they do not want to go through with the implantation process. Should these unwanted embryos be destroyed? Should they be used in experiments? Should they be offered to other couples? Who can decide what is to be done with them?

In respect to cryopreservation, some of the moral guidelines of the Church would be:

"Life must be protected with the utmost care from the moment of conception" (Vatican II, *Gaudium et Spes* 51)

"The freezing of embryos . . . constitutes an offense against the respect due to human beings . . ." (*Instruction on Respect for Human Life*, I. 6, Cong. Doctr. Faith, 1987).

"Respect for the dignity of the human being excludes all experimental manipulation of the human embryo" (*Charter of the Rights of the Family*, 4b, cited in *Instr. on Resp. for Human Life*, op.cit. I,4)

The safety of the IVF procedure has caused concern for some time now. Generally, the risks or hazards which were the object of concern had to do primarily with the possibility that the child so conceived would have a greater chance of acquiring a congenital abnormality. It was thought that the physical handling of the egg and the embryo before implantation would result in an increased rate of malformations. However, as reported recently by Dr. John D. Biggers, the experience to date with children already born does *not* bear out that fear. *Of course, it would not be surprising if some defects—physical or mental—would manifest themselves later, since this occurs even in normally conceived children.*

A more serious risk, of course, are the number of failures to implant. As one study indicated only 311 pregnancies resulted out of 2,864 embryos transferred to the uterine cavity; this means that over 2,553 human embryos were lost. How this number compares to the number lost as a result of natural conception is currently a controversial point.

Surrogate Parenting. In surrogate parenting, the woman is artificially inseminated by a man who is not her husband. She agrees to relinquish the child at birth to the man and his wife. A variation of this procedure is the situation in which the wife provides the egg and the husband the sperm. These are brought together in the laboratory. The resulting embryo is implanted, not in the woman who provided the egg but rather in another woman who accepts it and carries it to birth. Here again there is a prior agreement to give the child back to the parents. In the latter scenario, one could say that the child has two mothers: One is the woman who provided the egg (the "genetic mother") and the other is the "hired" woman, the "gestational mother."

There are many reasons for surrogate parenting besides infertility. A fertile woman may be unable to carry a child to term successfully. Or if the wife is a carrier of a serious genetic disease, the couple may decide to involve a surrogate mother. Finally, if the wife is engaged in a career that would be compromised if she were pregnant or took the time necessary for the proper birthing of a child, the couple may elect to have a child with the help of a surrogate mother.

These brief statements would be terrible incomplete without the mention of potential legal problems that may follow in the wake of surrogate parenting. Clearly, a written contract is important to lessen the potential legal complications. Some of the concerns include the following:

1) What if the surrogate mother refuses to relinquish the child at birth?
2) What does the surrogate mother do if the spouses changed their minds and did not want a child by this means?
3) What recourse is there if the surrogate mother wishes to abort the child, especially for reasons of health?
4) Who has the responsibility for the child born with severe abnormalities and rejected by both the couple and the surrogate mother?

These are thorny and painful problems for the couple and surrogate mother, but the impact on the child can be devastating.
192

Assisted Insemination[1]

Assisted Insemination, like the totally Artificial Insemination described above, can be described as follows: 1)It is a technique used to overcome problems such as oligospermia, vaginal secretions which react against semen, etc.; 2) It takes place when the woman is in the ovulatory phase of her cycle; and 3) It involves washing, centrifuging, and injecting the semen into the uterus. Unlike Artificial Insemination, Assisted Insemination involves no act of masturbation. Instead, the couple have complete intercourse, but most of the semen ejaculated in the act is retained in a "seminal receptacle," a condom-shaped covering for the penis, with a small perforation at the closed end so that some small amount of semen is actually deposited in the vagina. The seminal receptacle is especially designed to assist in infertility cases, and is made of silastic, a glass material which is processed so that it has even more elasticity than ordinary latex. Unlike latex, it is not injurious to sperm. Instead of using the silastic seminal receptacle, clinicians in some countries simply withdraw a large amount of semen with a syringe from the vagina after the couple's intercourse. Either the perforated seminal receptacle technique or the syringe technique means that marital intercourse, which the Church—and indeed the common sense of human beings—has always recognized as the substance of the authentic, humanly natural expression of conjugal love, is retained. Thus, many moralists maintain, the marital act remains the ultimate human source of any new life conceived, even though assistance is given to the insemination process.

Tubal Ovum Transfer With Sperm (TOTs)[2]

Dr. David McLaughlin slowly perfected this technique from 1983 to 1986 at St. Elizabeth's Catholic Hospital in Dayton, Ohio. The procedure is used to overcome certain fertility problems. First, the woman is stimulated to ovulation by injection of the proper hormones, and progress towards the moment of actual ovulation is monitored by pelvic ultrasound. On the proper day, a laparoscope tube is inserted to pick up an ovum from the now ripe ovary. Also semen is obtained and processed as in the Assisted Insemination methods discussed above. Semen and ovum are placed in a catheter, with a bubble of air separating them so that fertilization does not take place in this thin tube. The tube is then inserted into the fallopian tube and the gametes are flushed out. As the procedure has been refined over the past five years, success results have begun to surpass those of IVF. Moreover, it is a much less expensive process than IVF.

Gamete intro-Fallopian Transfer (GIFT)[3]

Dr. Ricardo Asch developed this technique at the University of Texas Health Center in Houston, Texas, to deal with so-called "mystery infertilities," that is, infertility for which no obstructed fallopian tubes or other obvious reason can be detected. It is similar to the TOT described above. However, as commonly practiced, the GIFT procedure does not obtain the male sperm from a conjugal act and is not performed in sequence to such an act. Hence Catholic moralists have reason to question whether GIFT can be morally acceptable unless it is modified to include these elements.

Conclusion

Technological reproduction is an attempt of modern human begins to meet the problem of infertility by means of technology. There are a wide variety of means available for this purpose but the next chapter will reflect on the morality of using these means.

Discussion Questions

1. List as many causes of male or female infertility as you can.
2. Why do some researchers use several ova for *in vitro* fertilization at the same time?
3. How large is the artificially fertilized embryo when implanted in the woman's uterus?
4. Is there any difference in moral significance between embryos lost in unsuccessful embryo transplant and embryos spontaneously aborted in normal pregnancies?
5. What two forms of surrogate parenting are described in this chapter?
6. Does *in vitro* fertilization remedy human infertility?

Notes

1. Lloyd Hess, PhD., "Assisting the Infertile Couple", in *Ethics and Medics*, February, 1986, pp. 2–4.
2. *Ibid.*, "TOTS is for Kids," in *Ethics and Medics*, Dec. 1988, pp 1–2.
3. *Ibid.*

Preview of
Chapter Seventeen

- This chapter focuses on the fact that technological reproduction threatens the dignity of children and parents and the integrity of the marital act.

- Every child has an equal and natural right to be conceived in the act of marital love which is a "natural sacrament." This guarantees the basis of an intimate interpersonal relationship with the parents.

- Every child-product of technology bears a handicap and is marked by a genuine privation in his or her own very personal identity or selfhood. Parents inflict this by deliberately using technology to satisfy their need of a child.

- The good motives and intentions of a childless couple do not alter the fact that they "produce" a child by non-marital acts and cause the fertilization of new human persons in a non-marital process.

- *In vitro* fertilization introduces further ethical liabilities beyond artificial insemination, subjecting human embryos to unjustifiable experimentation and, in some cases, to their deliberate destruction, if malformed.

CHAPTER 17

The Morality of Technological Reproduction

Introduction

The previous chapter ended with surrogate parenting through technological reproduction. An earlier kind of surrogate parenting, the process of adoption of children born out of wedlock, has always been morally acceptable. So has the practice of entrusting young children to nursemaids and nursery care. These represent acceptable forms of surrogate parenting, after birth.

Is technological surrogate parenting really different from the above? *In the light of Judeo-Christian sexual ethics outlined in this book and applied in this chapter, it is radically different.*

The previous chapter opened with a discussion of human infertility. After briefly mentioning therapeutic treatments to remedy this, it reviewed the current status of artificial insemination and *in vitro* fertilization. However, these ingenious techniques do not remedy infertility as such, rather they accomplish human fertilization through lesser or greater interventions of laboratory technology.

The child of technological intervention does not issue from normal human fertility and the procreative embrace of mother and father. This child's origin differs radically from the normal origin of a child who is later adopted or entrusted to a nursemaid.

Surrogate parenting through technological reproduction binds two women and a man into a triangle of human reproduction which violates the marriage covenant just as radically as the classical triangle in which the husband fathers a child from another woman than his wife. But in this form of technological reproduction the child suffers double jeopardy, both from the violation of marriage and from the substitution of a laboratory technique for an interpersonal procreative embrace.

Yet neither jeopardy looms as an irreversible moral evil in the secular sexual ethics outlined in Chapter 5. The two norms mentioned there, the free pursuit of sexual values as long as no other person is harmed, and the personal choice of sexual behavior by consenting adults, suggest that technological reproduction may be acceptable, "if no other person is harmed." *The handicap that should count as "harm" to the child-product of technology will be discussed below.*

The opening chapter of this book presented the Biblical teaching on human sexuality. It progressed from the *Genesis* vision of a man leaving father and mother to cling to his wife to the call in *Ephesians* that husbands love their wives with the *agapeic*, totally unselfish love that Christ has for the Church. The sexual ethics of the Bible not only offers no encouragement to technological reproduction, it pictures marriage as a totally interpersonal covenant; this is profoundly violated by impersonal technology.

This Biblical vision of human persons united in love and marriage by no means rules out research and technology for genuinely therapeutic purposes. But it asserts the inviolability of human persons themselves and of their interpersonal procreative embrace.

This book has focused on the twentieth century challenges in sexual ethics. Although technology has a long history, dating back to discovery of fire and the wheel, only in this century, has technology become applicable to the animal kingdom and, last of all, to human persons themselves. The tragedies of technologically efficient abortion and technologically efficient but dangerous and unsafe birth control pills indicate that technology can seductively subvert the dignity and moral integrity of human persons.

This chapter will reflect *first on the basic fact that technological reproduction threatens the dignity of children and parents and the integrity of the marital act.* Then it will address specifically *the newest reproductive technology, in vitro fertilization.*

The Child-Product of Technological Reproduction

Chapter 12 reviewed Biblical and Judeo-Christian teaching that a child is God's gift to parents, not the object of a right attached to the marriage covenant. Previously, Chapter 6 pointed out that Catholic teaching holds that God acts in a creative way through the procreative act of parents so that the newly conceived child enjoys a personal relationship to Him and an eternal destiny. Does this mean that God will not act through technological reproduction to give parents a child?

Evidently it does not. The 200 children mentioned in the last chapter are produced by *in vitro* fertilization are God's gift to their parents. We must presume that God acted creatively in their reproductive process since these children give every indication of enjoying the same personhood and personal relationship to God as the millions of children born through normal procreation each year.

But this in no way proves that technological reproduction is morally acceptable. Unmarried persons are able to procreate a child outside of marriage and family. This misuse of God's gift of procreativity is not morally good, but God tolerates it, lest human freedom—to do evil as well as good—be violated.

This moral reflection on technological reproduction can profitably begin with the child who is technologically reproduced and with his or her own rights. This consideration was alluded to in Chapter 6 with the reference to Fr. Ashley's argument that every child has a right to have "parents in the strict sense."[1]

It would seem unjust to discriminate against some children-to-be-born. Every child has a natural right to the fundamental security and self-identity that comes from one's generation through the "natural sacrament" of marital intercourse. This guarantees the child the basis for an intimate and meaningful interpersonal relationship with both parents who conceived the child in their interpersonal action which inherently is its own sign of mutual love, and love for the child.

Unfortunately, the parents do not always manifest love for each other in what God intends to be a conjugal act of love, and sometimes unmarried persons beget children as well. *But every child has an equal and natural right to be conceived in the act of conjugal love described in Chapter 6 as a "natural sacrament."*

Therefore, depending on the severity of the depersonalization attached to the particular type of technological reproduction employed, every child-product of technology bears a handicap, that is, a deprivation to some degree. The child is marked by a genuine privation in his or her own very personal identity or selfhood. Few people seem to recognize that technological reproduction unjustly begets handicapped children just as truly as procreation outside marriage unjustly deprives children of their right to be born from a relationship of lifelong love in marriage.

Obviously the handicap described here differs from a genetic defect like Down's syndrome or Tay-Sachs disease. Scientific studies have not so far shown any significant psychological impact this technological handicap makes on the lives of the child-products of technological reproduction. *But the personalist understanding of human life and procreation insists that this handicap is objectively present, whether or not it impacts measurable on the life-adjustment of these children.*

The impact seems to be serious, though less so, in the case of artificial insemination of the mother from the father. It expands with *in vitro* fertilization of the mother's ovum by the father's sperm. It expands considerably when a donor's sperm replaces that of the mother's husband and when donor's sperm is used with the mother's ovum for *in vitro* fertilization. The most radical handicap will undoubtedly occur when both donor sperm and donor ova are used to conceive children and, as it were, incubate them in a "rented womb" so they may subsequently be raised as children of the state or of some other adopting adult or group of adults.

This progression of increasingly serious handicaps to the child-product of technology may be dismissed by some as a merely theoretical "slippery slope," raising anxieties about slipping downward to ever more objectionable practices. Professional ethics are not easily impressed by the so-called "slippery slope" type of argument.

Yet because of the comparatively low pregnancy rate of AIH (artificial insemination from the husband), the slide down the slope to AID (artificial insemination from a donor) occurs rather easily. Likewise, while the initial IVF (*in vitro* fertilization) programs have assisted married couples, Dr. William G. Karow opened an Institute for IVF in Los Angeles in 1983 which expects to use surrogate wombs to carry IVF pregnancies.

But the force of this argument on behalf of the child does not rest uniquely on a "slippery slope" leading to ever greater handicaps to the children of technology. It rests on the basic injustice of parents who, to satisfy *their* need of a child, deliberately inflict a handicap on that child. Handicapped children are sometimes born through no fault of their parents, *but in this case the handicap is the direct result of technology deliberately used by the parents.* Hence even the well-meaning parents who use AIH have deprived their child unjustly of the full security and self-identity and interpersonal dependence on themselves that arises through conceiving a child in the "natural sacrament" of marital intercourse.

Admittedly the secular sexual ethics which heavily influences modern society gives little attention to this child-parent bonding through marital intercourse. Yet both secular and Christian humanists are now giving increasing attention to problems of ecology, problems which arise by disturbing fundamental relations in nature through technology. Christian humanists have a clearer vision of marriage and the family than their secular counterparts. Hence *they have a responsibility to proclaim the injustice done to the children of technology by altering one of the most fundamental relations in nature, that of child to parent.*

But the moral evaluation of technological reproduction can also be developed from the perspective of the parents and their actions in bringing children into existence through non-marital acts.

Parenthood by Non-Marital Acts

In Chapter 5 the view of the human person and human sexuality proposed after the Second Vatican Council by Popes Paul VI and John Paul II was described as an integrist personalism. In reference to sexuality this means accepting the unified body/spirit wholeness of conjugal activity and refusing to take apart the essential procreative and unitive meanings of the conjugal act.

One way of emphasizing this integration of all aspects of the total person into the conjugal act is to view it as having a single, unified *signification:* marital intercourse is designed by God to *express* a couple's calling to procreation *through* and *in* unitive love. Viewed this way each marital act should combine the procreative and unitive meanings of the marital relationship.

Chapter 10 reflected on the violence done to the marital act when its procreative potential is eliminated by contraception or sterilization. Technological reproduction, however, transfers that procreative potential to a non-marital context. The procreative gift marvelously written into the conjugal act is lifted from that context and manipulated through a series of non-marital acts of a technical nature.

In Both AIH and IVF where sperm and ovum come from a married couple with the intent of implanting the embryo in the wife's womb, the man and woman are married, but their acts are not marital acts. In the marital act of intercourse they signify and celebrate their total self-giving in love for each other. *In the acts of technological reproduction, even though they are married, their actions do not signify marriage or self-giving.*

In procreation by marital intercourse, one and the same act of choice, made by each spouse, governs both their sexual union and the procreation of the child. In technological reproduction a series of other acts are performed: Producing and collecting sperm, transferring sperm to uterus for artificial insemination, collecting ova if IVF is planned, mixing sperm and ova, implanting embryos for IVF, and the woman's act of choice to permit insemination or implantation.

Thus the child of technology does not come into existence as a gift flowing from an act expressive of marital union and as a new partner in the common life so vividly expressed by that act. Rather the child is conceived in the manner of a "product," the end product of a process carried out with the help of persons other than his or her parents.

Although childless couples may fervently wish for a child and fervently intend to treat the child as a person and not a product, *their motives and intentions do not change the nature of the process.* The very nature of that process bespeaks a product, a human product, the result of applied technology. The relationship of the technological child to the makers is one of radical inequality, of profound subordination. The child is handicapped because he or she *is* such a product, even if the child does not realize it. If the child knows his or her technological origin, he or she will consciously miss the security and self-identity of children conceived in an act of love in which both parents equally submitted themselves to each other and the source of life.[2]

Hence, technological reproduction by married couples is not merely objectionable because of a "slippery slope" to other uses of the technology outside marriage. *It already violates marriage in producing children by non-marital acts, even if it did not lead to other practices which violate marriage like the use of donor semen and donor ova.*

In normal parental procreation a child enters the community of the family, not as an object of production, but as a gift of God to be a kind of *partner* in the familial enterprise. Such a child has a *fundamental equality* with the parents. The community of the family receives a new member by a sacred act of *parental community*, the persons of husband and wife becoming "two in one flesh." Technological reproduction, both literally and symbolically, undermines the community of the family. Yet the new procedure of *in vitro* fertilization seems to have captivated the world's imagination and becomes a new fascination for obstetricians and gynecologists.

Specific Consideration of *In Vitro* Fertilization

The two moral reflections presented here, arguing against the production of handicapped children and the use of non-marital acts in technological reproduction, clearly apply to the new technique of *in vitro* fertilization.

Pope Pius XII rejected artificial insemination including AIH, in various addresses in the 1950's, precisely on the basis of the inseparability of these two meanings.[3] In anticipation of IVF Pope Pius XII said, "On the subject of the experiments in artificial human fecundation '*in vitro*', let it suffice for us to observe that they must be rejected as immoral *and absolutely* illicit."[4]

Pope John Paul II has strongly reaffirmed the teaching of Pope Paul VI on the inseparability of the two meanings of the conjugal act, the unitive and procreative meaning.[5]

Moreover, with his personal approval, the Vatican's Congregation for the Doctrine of the Faith in 1987 issued its *Instruction on Respect for Human life in its Origins and on the Dignity of Procreation*.[6] The document praised and encouraged scientific efforts to assist *the authentic conjugal act* of a couple to result in a pregnancy. It also warned, however, that any attempt to cause a pregnancy entirely without the authentic conjugal act's being substantially its cause would be an offense against sexuality itself as well as against the right of a child to be conceived out of married love and the sexual act which the Creator Himself has designed to express that love. At the same time, the Instruction admits that in some cases it is not easy to see whether a particular scientific procedure is legitimately aiding the authentic conjugal act itself to achieve a pregnancy, and when, to the contrary, the procedure is displacing the conjugal act. The Vatican document, however, clearly rejects IVF procedures of any kind whatsoever, even involving gametes taken from a husband and wife. *A fortiori* it rejects any IVF procedure in which a wife is impregnated with either a sperm or ovum from a person outside her marriage.

The document also rejects any experimentation on or destruction of embryos or fetuses purely for clinical or scientific purposes, and points out that IVF creates precisely this temptation and opportunity. The warning was prophetic. Only two years later information surfaced that reproductive clinicians were indeed deliberately causing multiple pregnancies in a woman, and then killing off all but one or two living embryos in the process of "reduction" which we have described in the previous chapter.

The Instruction reiterates, then, the Church's constant criteria regarding "respect for human life" and "the dignity of procreation", and rejects certain procedures which clearly offend against these criteria. At the same time, the Instruction invites further thought and discussion of these and other procedures possible for the future. It teaches that if "a technical meals facilitates the conjugal act or helps it reach its natural objectives, it can be morally acceptable." It does not explicitly approve assisted insemination or TOTS as described in this chapter. Catholic moralists who believe these are legitimate forms of assisting the marital act would like to see an explicit approval. In the absence of such approval, they can only point to their judgment of the "solid probability" that these procedures are acceptable. In moral theology, "solid probability" means that the arguments for the moral acceptability of a particular practice are respectable defensible within the context of Catholic doctrine, unless and until the Church officially rejects them. Catholics who are in doubt about an issue may in good conscience guide their decisions by these "solidly probable opinions."

Furthermore, IVF introduces another serious ethical liability beyond the objections to artificial insemination. For tiny human beings become the subjects of an experimental procedure. The previous chapter noted that experience to date has not shown an increased rate of malformations among IVF babies. But future defects may still appear, as they often appear in subsequently in normally conceived children. And, of course, the child may well by psychologically scarred if it is discovered that the parents had agreed to abortion if the child was not perfectly normal.

In the case of IVF, who has the right to subject these tiny human subjects to the experimental process of laboratory fertilization? Paul Ramsey has argued strongly that IVF should be considered unethical experimentation on a human subject unless the possibility of irreparable damage to this child-to-be can be definitively excluded.[7] Notice here that the harm to the child may well be physiologically or psychologically very obvious, as opposed to the more subtle handicap described above as afflicting every child of technology because he or she was conceived a non-marital act. Is it possible that parents who have artificially produced a child will be more likely to "manhandle" their product as it grows up?

Statistics in the previous chapter noted that 2,553 human embryos were lost in the course of achieving 311 IVF pregnancies. The companion volume to this one, *A Handbook on Critical Life Issues*, discussed the beginning of human life.[8] It concluded with the Second Vatican Council that "Life must be protected with the utmost care from the moment of conception." *This means that tiny human embryos must not be destroyed or experimented upon,* even though some philosophers speculate about a delayed infusion of the spiritual soul.[9]

How many embryos were so far actually destroyed in IVF by deliberate action, perhaps because they were imperfect, and how many were lost because the procedure of implantation was simply unsuccessful cannot be determined. If the procedure itself cannot be morally justified, this further implication simply adds to the moral objections to the procedure.

On the other hand, some experts in ethics within the Catholic community have defended AIH and are also willing to justify IVF if: It can be limited to married couples, be proven comparatively safe for the child produced, and deliberate wastage of embryos can be excluded. Those who adopt the method of ethical proportionalism described in Chapter 6 are open to considering that instances of technological reproduction in marriage may be described as containing only ontic or premoral evil.[10] The editors of this book have not accepted that methodology although they are most sympathetic to the burden of childlessness.

Hence, while IVF in marriage appeals to all who support and encourage family life because a child is produced, *the moral objections outlines in this chapter cannot be readily overcome.* The procedure may become relatively common in the future, much as contraception and sterilization have. But this will more likely indicate the persuasiveness of the current secular sexual ethics rather than the compatibility of IVF with Catholic teaching.

Future scientific developments that are fully compatible with Catholic teaching can be expected. This would include more successful repair of blocked Fallopian tubes and even possibly replacement of such tubes as well as other methods to make sure the woman's ova are available for fertilization in the at of conjugal intercourse. Even now the teaching of Pope Pius XII does not rule out assistance in the conjugal act of insemination.[11]

Conclusion

This chapter has raised serious moral objections to the technological reproduction of human persons. An earlier chapter (10) objected to the technology of contraception and sterilization. In both cases the moral argument rests on respect for the nature of the human person and his or her acts of conjugal intercourse. The integrist personalism of Pope John Paul II is not anti-technology but pro-person.

Paul Ramsey has written that humans ought not to play God before they learn to be humans, and after they learn to be humans they will not play God.[12] The approach to critical sexual issues presented in this volume uses Biblical wisdom and Church teaching to help men and women learn how to be authentic sexual persons and to express authentic conjugal love. In a sinful world this ideal will never be fully realized, but it beckons all who believe that "God is love and he who abides in love abides in God." (I Jn. 4:16)

Discussion Questions

1. How does the Biblical teaching on sexuality oppose technological reproduction?
2. Why does every child have an equal and natural right to be conceived in the act of conjugal love?
3. How can one say that technological reproduction begets handicapped children?
4. What is a "slippery slope" argument? Is it the only argument against technological reproduction?
5. What is wrong with parents having children through non-marital acts?
6. What serious ethical liability does IVF introduce over and above the objections to artificial insemination?
7. What future developments in medical science can be expected which will remedy infertility without resorting to technological reproduction?

Notes
1. Ashley, Benedict M., "A Child's Right to His Own Parents: A Look at Two Value Systems," *Hospital Progress*, 61 (Aug., 1980) pp. 17–49.
2. Cf. "*In Vitro* Fertilization: Morality and Public Policy" a statement submitted to the British Government Committee of Inquiry into Human Fertilization and Embryology by the Joint Committee on Bio-Ethical Issues of the Catholic Bishops of Great Britain, Mar. 2, 1983. See also, May, William E., "Artful Childmaking: Reproduction or Procreation?" *Homiletic and Pastoral Review*, May, 1982, pp. 24–32 and 43–46.
3. CF. especially the address of Pope Pius XII to the Second World Congress on Fertility and Sterility on May 19, 1956, *The Pope Speaks*, 3:2, Autumn, 1956, pp 191–197.
4. *Ibid*, p. 194.
5. *The Apostolic Exhortation on the Family (Familiaris Consortio)* Nov. 22, 1981, Vatican Text. #32.
6. *Origins*, March 19, 1987, vol. 16: no. 40
7. May, *op.cit.*, pp. 29–31.
8 . Edited by Donald G. McCarthy and Edward J. Bayer, (St. Louis: Pope John Center, 1982), Chapters 7–9, pp. 79–119.
9. See *Declaration on Abortion* of the Sacred Congregation for the Doctrine of the Faith, Nov. 18, 1974, especially #12–13 and footnote 19.
10. See, for example, Keane, Philip S., *Sexual Morality: A Catholic Perspective* (NY: Paulist Press, 1977), p. 140.
11. See, for example, O'Donnell, Thomas, *Medicine and Christian Morality*, (NY: Alba House, 1976) p. 269.
12. Ramsey, Paul, *Fabricated Man*, (New Haven, CT, Yale U. Press, 1970), p. 138.

Bibliography

The following books offer further resource material on the themes of this Handbook. They were selected as representative of the Judeo-Christian tradition and Catholic teaching.

Pope John Paul II, Apostolic Exhortation on the Role of the Christian Family in the Modern World, Familiaris Consortio (Boston: St. Paul Editions, 1981.)

Pope John Paul II, Original Unity of Man and Women, (Boston: St. Paul Editions, 1981).

Ashley, O.P., Benedict M. and O'Rourke O.P., Kevin D., Health Care Ethics, A Theological Analysis. St. Louis, MO: Catholic Health Assoc. of U.S., 2nd Edit., 1982.

Atkinson, Gary M., and Moraczewski, O.P., Albert S., editors, Genetic Counseling, the Church, and the Law. St. Louis, MO: The Pope John Center, 1980.

Atkinson, Gary M., and Moraczewski, O.P., Albert S., A Moral Evaluation of Contraception and Sterilization, St. Louis, MO: The Pope John Center, 1979.

Billings, Evelyn, and Westmore, Anna, The Billings Method. Victoria, Australia: O'Donovan, 1980.

Cavanagh, John R., Counseling the Homosexual, Huntington, IN: Our Sunday Visitor Inc., 1977.

Gratsch, Edward, editor, Principles of Catholic Theology, A Synthesis of Dogma and Morals, Staten Island, NY: Alba House, 1981.

Human Body: Papal Teachings, Boston, MA, Daughters of St. Paul, 1960.

Human Sexuality and Personhood, St. Louis, MO: The Pope John Center, 1981.

Kipley, John F. and Shella, The Art of Natural Family Planning, Cincinnati, OH: The Couple to Couple League International, 1979.

Love and Sexuality: Official Catholic Teachings, Wilmington, NC, McGrath Publ. Co: a Consortium Book, 1976.

May, William E., Editor, Principles of Catholic Moral Life, Chicago, IL: Franciscan Herald Press, 1980.

May, William E., Human Existence, Medicine, and Ethics, Chicago, IL: Franciscan Herald Press, 1977.

May William E., Sex, Marriage, and Chastity, Chicago, IL: Franciscan Herald Press, 1981.

McCarthy, Donald G., and Bayer, Edward J., Handbook on Critical Life Issues, St. Louis, MO: The Pope John Center, 1982.

Moraczewski, O.P., Albert S., editor, Genetic Medicine and Engineering, Ethical and Social Dimensions, St. Louis, MO: The Catholic Health Association Publications, 1983, in press.

New Technologies of Birth and Death, St. Louis, MO: The Pope John Center, 1980.

Noonan, John T., Contraception: A History of Its Treatment by the Catholic Theologians and Canonists, Cambridge, MA, Belknap, 1965.

O'Donnell, S. J., Thomas J., Medicine and Christian Morality, Staten Island, NY: Alba, House, 1976.

Ramsey, Paul, Fabricated Man, The Ethics of Genetic Control, New Haven, CT: Yale University Press, 1970.

Schillebeeckx, Edward, Marriage: Human Reality and Saving Mystery, 2 vols., New York, NY: 1965.

Wakenfield, John, Artful Childmaking, Artificial Insemination in Catholic Teaching, St. Louis, MO: The Pope John Center, 1978.

Index

Goods (of marriage), 17
Grace, 83, 90
Gradualness, law of, 125
Gratian, 19
Greeks, 162
Guitton, Jean, 99

Handbooks (for priest-confessors), 13, 20
Hannah, 141
Happiness, 2, 9
Häring, Bernard, 30
Harvey, John 166
Health care ethics, 66
Heart, 8, 110
Hemophilia, 135
Herpes, 110
Hilgers, Dr., 97
Holiness (interior), 7–9
Holmes, Oliver Wendell, 45
Holy. *See* Sacred
Holy Spirit. *See* Spirit, Holy
Homosexual actions, 4, 48, 57, 59, 65, 70
Homosexuality, 160–169, 171–183
Hope, 90
Human (to be), 141
Hunter, John, 185
Hysterectomy, 112

Image of God, 4, 16, 51, 61
Immorality, 8, 14
Implants, contraceptive. *See* Depo-Provera
Impurity, moral, 8, 31 ff
Impurity, ritual, 14
Incest, 5
Indissolubility (of marriage) 83–84, 102
Individualism, radical, 65
Infant mortality, 130
Infection, contraceptive. *See* Depo-Provera
Infertility, 184, 186–187
Information, right to, 146–147
Inherent evil. *See* Intrinsic evil
Innocence, 6
Insanity, 29
Insemination, artificial, 33
Institutiones, 26–28
Intentions, 8
Intercourse, 10, 12, 14, 15, 16, 18, 19
Interior (disposition), 10
Interior holiness. *See* Holiness
Inter-personal relationship, 64
Intimacy, 4

Intrauterine device, 106, 108, 109, 111, 113
Intrinsic evil, 31
In vitro fertilization (IVF), 33, 140, 145–146, 184, 187–190, 195, 202–204
Involvement (in world), 11, 15–17
Israel. *See* Jews
Ius in Corpus. See *Jus in Corpus*

Jacob, 4
Jerusalem (Council of), 6
Jesus Christ, 6–10, 15, 82, 99, 141–143, 197
Jewish Scriptures. *See* Old Testament
Jews, 3–7, 162
Jews, Eastern European. *See* Askenazi
Jorgensen, Christine, 156
Joseph (son of Jacob), 5
Judeo-Christian tradition, 4, 15
Jus in Corpus, 84
Justice. *See* Rights
Justification, 7

Kant, Immanuel, 42
Karlen, Arlo, 162
Karow, William G., 199
Keane, Philip S., 72
Kelly, Gerard, 30
Kinsey studies, 162, 164, 165, 166
Kippley, John and Sheila, 96, 102
Knaus, Dr., 96

Lambeth Conference, 47, 96
Language, sexual acts as, 60, 101
Law of love, 6
Le Maistre, Martin, 20, 25
Lesbians, 162
Liberalism, doctrinal, 46
Life expectancy, 38
Liguori. *See* Alphonsus Liguori, St.
Lipid, 132
Literalism, 46
Liturgy (of wedding), 20, 24
Liver tumors, 110
Love, 3, 7, 8, 13, 17, 20, 30, 31, 56, 57 67 69, 85, 91
Lust, 8
Luther, Martin, 26

Marriage, 2, 3, 4, 6
Marriage, canonically valid, 155

214

Pope John Center Publications

The Pope John XXIII Medical-Moral Research and Education Center has dedicated itself to approaching current and emerging medical-moral issues from the perspective of Catholic teaching and the Judeo-Christian heritage. Publications of the Pope John Center include:

CRITICAL ISSUES IN CONTEMPORARY HEALTH CARE (Proceedings of the 1989 Bishops' Workshop). Edited by Russell E. Smith. $17.95.
This book centers around the general theme of health care and its technologies. Among the specific topics treated are: euthanasia, the right to die movements, pastoral considerations of life and death issues, ethics committees in health care facilities, fetal and newborn tissue transplânts, psychosexual maturity, Catholic identity and hospital mergers, moral issues in the artificial provision of nutrition and hydration, and teaching moral theology in the contemporary world.

REPRODUCTIVE TECHNOLOGIES, MARRIAGE AND THE CHURCH (Proceedings of the 1988 Bishops' Workshop), 318 pp., $17.95.
This book provides a commentary on and a discussion of the Vatican's *Instruction on Respect for Human Life in its Origin and on the Dignity of Procreation* (1987). Topics covered range from an overview of current magisterial teaching regarding procreation to a consideration of the values presupposed by reproductive technologies, an update on AIDS, and suggestions for pastoral applications of the Church's teaching on human procreation and sexual diseases.

THE AIDS CRISIS AND THE CONTRACEPTIVE MENTALITY by Msgr. Orville N. Griese, S.T.D., J.C.D., and Dr. Eugene F. Diamond with a Pastoral Commentary by The Most Reverend Donald W. Montrose, 1988, 69 pp., $3.95.
A moral evaluation of potential means of protecting the general population from the scourge of AIDS . . . Using the AIDS crisis to renew dedication to Christian standards of morality.

SEXUALITY: THEOLOGICAL VOICES—Kevin T. McMahon $14.95.
A Critical Analysis of American Catholic Theological Thought from 1965 through 1980.

THEOLOGIANS AND AUTHORITY WITHIN THE LIVING CHURCH by Msgr. James J. Mulligan, 1986, 139 pp., $13.95.
The author's intention is to answer some questions that have been raised about the proper place of authority and theology in the Catholic Church. Using clear and readable language, the author seeks to explain, to clarify and to share with the reader a context within which he thinks there can be peace.

CATHOLIC IDENTITY IN HEALTH CARE By Msgr. Orville N. Griese, S.T.D., J.C.D., 1987, 537 pp., $17.95.
This book is a detailed commentary on the *Ethical and Religious Directives for Catholic Health Facilities* approved by the National Confer-

ence of Catholic Bishops. The author organized his material around nine core principles upon which the *Directives* rest.

SCARCE MEDICAL RESOURCES AND JUSTICE (Proceedings of the 1987 Bishops' Workshop). $17.95.
These are the Proceedings of the 1987 Bishops' Workshop in which, with the help of appropriate experts, the bishops pondered the respective responsibilities of individuals and various institutions with regards to the equitable distribution of burdens and benefits in the provision of health care.

CONSERVING HUMAN LIFE (The Pope John Center Edition) by The Most Reverend Daniel A. Cronin, $17.95.
Originally written in 1958 before the issue had become emotionally charged, this updated and edited version of a doctoral dissertation traces the development of the Church's understanding of the moral law in regard to the ordinary and extraordinary means of conserving life. With Commentaries. 1989.

THE FAMILY TODAY AND TOMORROW: The Church Addresses Her Future (Proceedings of the 1985 Bishops' Workshop) Edited by Donald G. McCarthy, Ph.D., 1985, 291 pp., $17.95.
One of the family's fundamental tasks is: "to build up the kingdom of God in history by participating in the life and mission of the Church" (Familiaris Consortio, 49). The challenges and obstacles that inhibit the family in this role today are examined, with reflections from the Church's teachings and possible future directions. Fifteen experts in sociology, psychology, medicine and theology have contributed to this volume.

THEOLOGIES OF THE BODY: Humanist and Christian By Benedict M. Ashley, O.P., 1985, 770 pp., $20.95.
With a rare breadth of vision and insightful erudition, this wide ranging theological study of human materiality compares and contrasts two world viewpoints—the humanist and the Christian. It is an historical, philosophical and theological approach to a non-dualistic anthropology as a foundation for Christian ethics.

MORAL THEOLOGY TODAY: Certitudes and Doubts (Proceedings of the 1984 Bishops' Workshop) 1984, 355 pp., $17.95.
This book presents a concise survey of morals and ethics in their biblical and systematic theology roots, their historical development, and the relationships of theologians to bishops, the tradition and the magisterium. Contemporary challenges in moral methodologies are examined and compared with traditional principles of exceptionless moral norms, totality, double-effect and the moral inseparability of the unitive and procreative meanings of the conjugal act.

SEX AND GENDER: A Theological and Scientific Inquiry Edited by Mark Schwartz, Sc.D., Albert S. Moraczewski, OP, Ph.D. and James A. Monteleone, MD, 1983, 385 pp., $19.95.
This is an attempt to provide in the area of human sexuality the most current scientific data and additional psychological, philosophical and theological reflections upon that data from the viewpoint of the meanings of sexuality as expressed in Catholic teaching.

TECHNOLOGICAL POWERS AND THE PERSON: Nuclear Energy and Reproductive Technologies (Proceedings of the 1983 Bishops' Workshop) 1983, 500 pp., $15.95.
In the 1983 Dallas workshop, the assembled bishops listened, pondered and reacted to scientific and theological experts speaking on the awesome powers of nuclear energy (for peaceful purposes) and reproductive technologies. This book is a collection of the lectures and edited discussions.

HANDBOOK ON CRITICAL SEXUAL ISSUES Edited by Donald G. McCarthy, Ph.D. and Edward J. Bayer, S. T. D., Revised edition, 1989, 220 pp., $9.95.
Taking an historical approach beginning with biblical roots of Catholic teaching developing through early and medieval periods and bringing it up to post Vatican II, the book attempts to present the roots of sexual norms in Catholic sexual teaching. After discussing the Christian vocation of marriage and natural family planning, the book enters into the second part in which specific sexual issues are considered.

HANDBOOK ON CRITICAL LIFE ISSUES Edited by Donald G. McCarthy, Ph.D. and Edward J. Bayer, S.T.D., Revised edition, 1989. 220 pp., $9.95.
This is a carefully edited version of the presentation made by thirty-one experts in medicine, theology, psychology, law and sociology who for twelve days addressed such issues as abortion, defective fetal development, organ transplants, technology for prolongation of life, and brain-related criterion for the determination of a person's death.

MORAL RESPONSIBILITY IN PROLONGING LIFE DECISIONS Edited by Donald G. McCarthy, Ph.D. and Albert S. Moraczewski, OP, Ph.D., 1982, 316 pp., $9.95.
This book contains twenty chapters plus two appendices and discusses the medical, moral and legal aspects of prolonging life decisions. It also examines the specific responsibilities of administrators of health care facilities, physicians, nurses and pastoral care persons.

HUMAN SEXUALITY AND PERSONHOOD (Proceedings of the 1981 Bishops' Workshop) 1981, 254 pp., $9.95.
With input from several relevant scientific disciplines, this Bishops' Workshop sought to present a contemporary and balanced theology of human sexuality and marriage in the light of magisterial teaching and a Christian theology of the human person.

GENETIC COUNSELING: The Church and the Law Edited by Gary Atkinson, Ph.D., and Albert S. Moraczewski, OP, Ph.D., 1980, 259 pp., $9.95.
An appreciative review in the December 1980 issue of *Theological Studies* (Page 805) describes succinctly: "Highly recommended for genetic counselors, pastors, and students. Its clear common succinct style makes the book a good introduction to biogenetic morality and a valuable survey of the present debate."

NEW TECHNOLOGIES OF BIRTH AND DEATH: Medical, Legal, and Moral Dimensions (Proceedings of the 1980 Bishops' Workshop) 1980, 196 pp., $8.95.

Five theologians, two physicians and two lawyers discuss subjects as old as abortion and contraception and as new as in vitro fertilization and the ovulation method of family planning. The book also reviews efforts to· determine if human death has occurred even though vital signs are artificially maintained.

A MORAL EVALUATION OF CONTRACEPTION AND STERILIZATION: A Dialogical Study by Gary Atkinson, Ph.D. and Albert S. Moraczewski, OP, Ph.D., 1980, 115 pp., $4.95.

The authors of this paper hope it will be a contribution to a more clear understanding of the multifaceted issues of contraception by presenting accurately, clearly, and fairly the principal arguments of this controversy.

ARTFUL CHILDMAKING: Artificial Insemination in Catholic Teaching by John C. Wakefield, Ph.D., 1978, 205 pp., $8.95.

By providing an historical and theological review of the Church's teaching with regard to artificial insemination, the present publication does some of the ground work for an understanding of the Catholic Church's position with regards to technological reproduction.

AN ETHICAL EVALUATION OF FETAL EXPERIMENTATION Edited by Donald G. McCarthy, Ph.D. and Albert S. Moraczewski, OP, Ph.D., 1976, 137 pp., $8.95.

The present study seeks to analyze the ethical issues involved in fetal experimentation and to discover the valid foundations for a broadly based consensus concerning our need as a human, civilized community to protect the fetus. The book also includes a detailed discussion of the issue of delayed hominization and its refutation.

The following books have been published collaboratively with the Catholic Health Association of the United States:

GENETIC MEDICINE AND ENGINEERING: Ethical and Social Dimensions Edited by Albert S. Moraczewski, OP, Ph.D., 1983, 198 pp., $17.50.

This book intends to assist the decision-makers in Catholic Health Ministries, especially in forming appropriate and practical policies in matter concerning these developing technologies in the area of genetic medicine and engineering. It is a collection of articles by experts in the field of genetics and ethics.

ETHICS COMMITTEES: A Challenge for Catholic Health Care Edited by Sister Margaret John Kelly, D.C., Ph.D. and Donald G. McCarthy, Ph.D., 1984, 151 pp., $15.50.

This work treats the various needs which have contributed to the development of the Ethics Committees; reflect on ethical methodologies and legal aspects of such committees and offers models for various types of ethics committees to meet the needs at the institutional, diocesan and multi-institutional system levels.

219

DETERMINATION OF DEATH: Theological, Medical, Ethical and Legal Issues by Albert S. Moraczewski, OP, Ph.D. and J. Stuart Showalter, JD, MFS, St. Louis, The Catholic Health Association of the U.S. 1982, 39 pp., $2.50.

In a concise manner, this work focuses on the question, "Is the Patient Dead?" In the first section, the biblical and theological roots of the concept of person and the philosophical aspects of life and death are briefly reviewed. In the final section, the statutory and case law aspects are discussed.

As a service to those interested in the meaning of "moral" laws and norms, The Pope John Center is making available a published doctoral dissertation:

THE MEANING OF THE TERM "MORAL" IN ST. THOMAS AQUINAS by Brian Thomas Mullady, OP, S. T. D., Pontifical Academy of St. Thomas, looks squarely at some of the contemporary issues especially with regards to the denial of exceptionless moral norms. $12.00.

These books may be ordered from: The Pope John Center, 186 Forbes Road, Braintree, MA 02184, Telephone (617) 848–6965. Prepayment is encouraged. Please add $2.00 for shipping and handling for the first book ordered and $1.00 for each additional book.

Subscriptions to the Pope John Center monthly newsletter, *ETHICS AND MEDICS,* may be sent to the same address.